student manual of physical examination

student manual of physical examination

Marie Scott Brown, R.N., M.S., Ph.D.
Associate Professor, Parent-Child Nursing, School of Nursing
University of Colorado Medical Center, Denver

Carolyn M. Hudak, R.N., M.S.
Associate Professor of Nursing, School of Nursing
Assistant Professor of Medicine, School of Medicine
University of Colorado Medical Center, Denver

Janice Brenneman, R.N., M.S.
Assistant Professor, School of Nursing
University of Colorado Medical Center, Denver

Kathleen Walsh, R.N., M.S.N.
Associate Director, Nursing Service; Assistant Professor, School of Nursing
University of Colorado Medical Center, Denver

Karen M. Kleeman, R.N., M.S.
Assistant Professor, School of Nursing
University of Maryland, College Park

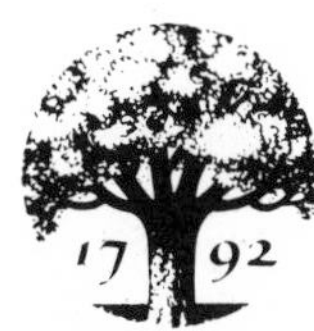

J. B. Lippincott Company
Philadelphia
New York / San Jose / Toronto

Copyright © 1977 by J. B. Lippincott Company

This book is fully protected by copyright and, with the exception of brief excerpts for review, no part of it may be reproduced in any form, by print, photoprint, microfilm, or any other means, without written permission from the publisher.

Distributed in Great Britain by Blackwell Scientific Publications, Oxford, London, and Edinburgh

ISBN 0-397-54211-9

Library of Congress Catalog Card Number 77-13693

Printed in the United States of America
1 3 5 7 9 8 6 4 2

Library of Congress Cataloging in Publication Data

Main entry under title:

Student manual of physical examination.

Bibliography: p.
1. Physical diagnosis. 2. Nursing. I. Brown, Marie Scott.
RT48.S78 616.07'54 77-13693
ISBN 0-397-54211-9

contributing authors

The original work for certain chapters in this book was written by three nurse practitioners. Although this original work has since gone through several revisions, we would like to credit the following people:

Carol Campbell—for the original draft of the cardiovascular system section
Carla Littlefield—for the original draft of the eye section
Maureen Collar—for the original draft of the nose, mouth, and throat section

introduction

This student manual was developed as part of a project to incorporate primary care concepts into the undergraduate and graduate curricula at the University of Colorado School of Nursing. The pilot text was used by a number of nurse practitioner students and incoming graduate students and was revised as a result of these experiences. The design of the manual allows the student to do as much preliminary work as possible, with the result that expensive resources such as faculty time and/or clinic or preceptor time are conserved.

The individual sections on specific parts of the physical examination are similar in format. The sections are divided into areas that deal with *basic knowledge, inspection, palpation, percussion,* and *auscultation.* Each of these areas has its own objectives, learning activities, and definitions, and is followed by a set of review questions. A self-evaluation key is provided at the end of each section so that the student can monitor his progress. The required materials for each section are outlined at the beginning of the section.

This manual can be used in a core course that teaches examination of the adult, the pregnant woman, and the child. It can be used by students taking a course in only one of these areas by simply deleting those parts of the material that pertain to other age groups. The book is constructed so that portions may be detached.

We wish to express sincere thanks to the individuals who helped in the development of these materials and especially to the students who used them and gave us valuable feedback so that the course content could be refined into a useful learning tool. We are especially grateful to Linda Perkins for her many efforts in the preparation of this material.

Marie Scott Brown
Carolyn M. Hudak
Janice K. Brenneman
Kathleen A. Walsh
Karen M. Kleeman

contents

1

physical examination: general approach, methods of examination, and clinical measurements

TO THE STUDENT

The format described in the Introduction will be followed in this and all succeeding sections of the manual. This first section presents the general approaches to the physical examination of both children and adults. The five methods of examination (inspection, palpation, percussion, auscultation, and smelling) will be discussed. Although there are eight important clinical measurements (height, weight, head and chest circumference, pulse, respiration, blood pressure, and temperature) and the student is expected to be able to list all eight of these at this time, only two (height and weight) will be discussed in this section. Head and chest circumference will be treated in the section on the face, head, and neck.

Recommended materials:

1 Alexander, Mary, and Brown, Marie. *Pediatric Physical Diagnosis for Nurses.* New York: McGraw-Hill Book Co., 1974

2 Bates, Barbara. *A Guide to Physical Examination.* Philadelphia: J. B. Lippincott Co., 1974

3 a clinical scale with a device for measuring height
4 an infant scale
5 an infant measuring board
6 access to two adults and two infants who will allow you to examine them

BASIC KNOWLEDGE

Behavioral Objectives

The student will be able to:

1 list the categories of the body to be examined when doing a physical examination according to this categorization: general survey; vital signs; skin; head; eyes; ears; nose and sinus; mouth and pharynx; cranial nerves; neck; back; posterior thorax; breasts and axillae; anterior thorax and lungs; heart; abdomen; inguinal area; genitalia and rectal exam; extremities; musculoskeletal system; peripheral vascular system
2 list the five methods of examination: inspection, palpation, percussion, auscultation, and smelling
3 list the eight commonly used clinical measurements: height, weight, head circumference, chest circumference, pulse, respiration, blood pressure, and temperature
4 state in writing how to convert kilograms to pounds and pounds to kilograms
5 correctly weigh an adult on a scale
6 state in writing how to convert centimeters to inches and inches to centimeters
7 measure the height of an adult on a height measuring device
8 measure the length of an infant on a measuring board
9 plot the weight of an infant or child over three on an appropriate graph and state in writing the percentile on which the child falls
10 accurately plot the height of an infant or child over three on an appropriate graph and state in writing the percentile on which the child falls
11 answer the review questions for this section
12 describe the general appearance of a person and record the findings
13 prepare a person psychologically and emotionally for a physical examination.

Learning Activities

Required

A *Read:*
Alexander and Brown, Bates

B *Weigh:* (1) two adults on a scale. Convert the pound measurement to kilograms
(2) two infants on a scale. Convert the pound measurement to kilograms and plot this weight on the appropriate graph. State what percentile the child's weight falls on.

C *Measure:* two adults with a height-measuring device. Convert the feet and inches to centimeters.

D *Observe:* two infants and adults and record your observations in one short, succinct phrase (i.e., "a three-month-old, white, alert infant").

Review Questions

WORD CHOICE

(Underline the correct word or words)

Adult and Pediatric

1 Of the five methods of examination, the most important is (inspection; palpation; percussion; auscultation; smelling).

2 The (fingertips; backs of the fingers; palms) are most sensitive to fine tactile details.
3 The (fingertips; backs of the fingers; palms) are most sensitive to temperature.
4 Such qualities as moisture, pulsatility, crepitus, and texture should be appreciated through (inspection; palpation; percussion; auscultation; smelling).

Pediatric

5 With a good explanation, the ear and throat examination is seldom threatening to a child (18–22 months; 22–26 months; 3 years or older).
6 The child most likely to be frightened during a physical examination is (an infant; a two-year-old; a four-year-old; an adolescent).
7 The age at which a child is most likely to protest when placed on the examining table is (6 weeks; 4 months; 6–8 months).

Self-Evaluation Key

REVIEW QUESTIONS (p. 2)

1. inspection
2. fingertips
3. back of fingers
4. palpation
5. 3 years or older
6. a 2-year-old
7. 6–8 months

2

skin and lymphatic system

TO THE STUDENT

The examination of the skin and lymphatic system is usually incorporated into the general system of the physical examination.

Recommended materials:

1 Alexander, Mary, and Brown, Marie. *Pediatric Physical Diagnosis for Nurses.* New York: McGraw-Hill Book Co., 1974

2 Bates, Barbara. *A Guide to Physical Examination.* Philadelphia: J. B. Lippincott Co., 1974

3 Blue Hill Educational Systems, Inc. *Pediatric Physical Examination—General Appearance, Skin, Lymph, Head, Face and Neck* (Videotape: 48 minutes)

4 Blue Hill Educational Systems, Inc. *Physical Assessment Examinations—Integument/Lymph Nodes* (Videotape: 18 minutes)

5 access to three adults and three children who will allow you to examine their skin and lymphatic systems

BASIC KNOWLEDGE: SKIN

Behavioral Objectives

The student will be able to:

1 define in writing the terms listed under *Definitions*

2 answer in writing all *Review Questions*

3 label the accompanying figures of the skin layers and the nail

4 state in writing that examination of the skin includes inspection and palpation in good lighting.

Learning Activities

I Required

A *Read:*

Alexander and Brown, Bates

B *Label:* Figures 2–1 and 2–2

II Optional

See listing of additional references and materials specific to skin and lymph in *Bibliography*.

Figure 2–1
Skin

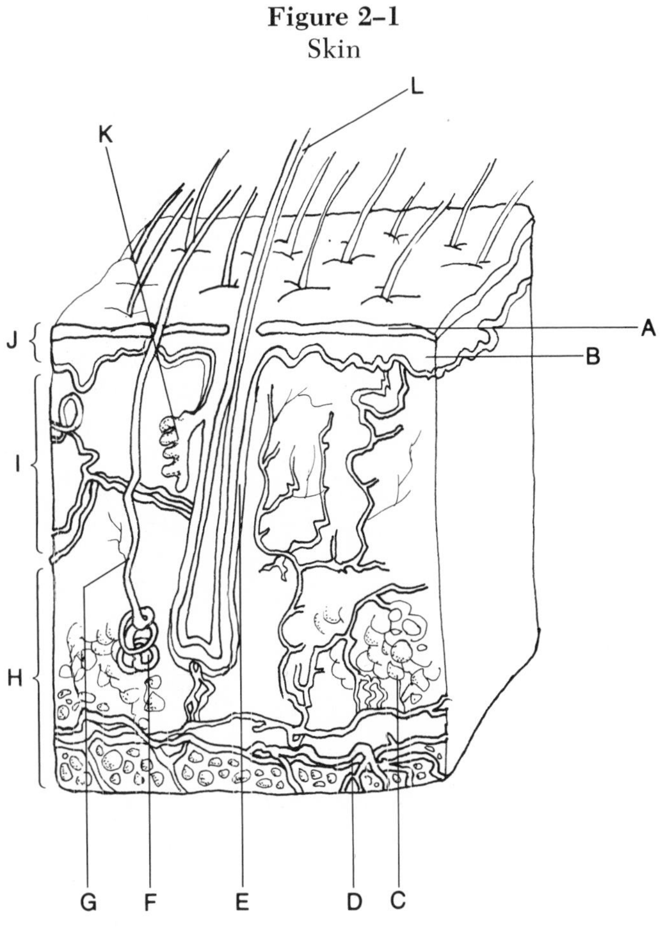

Label:

_____1. **epidermis**	_____7. **cellular layer of epidermis**
_____2. **horny layer of epidermis**	_____8. **dermis**
_____3. **subcutaneous tissue**	_____9. **fat**
_____4. **hair**	_____10. **duct of sweat gland**
_____5. **hair follicle**	_____11. **sweat gland**
_____6. **sebaceous gland**	_____12. **blood vessel**

Figure 2–2
Skin

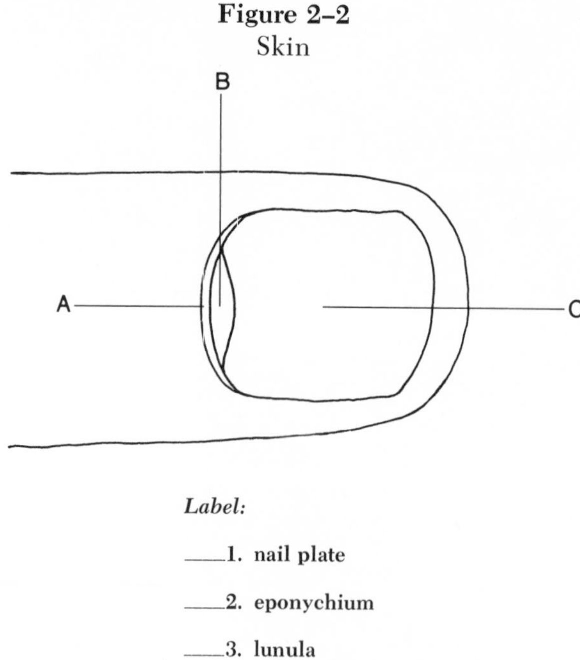

Label:

____1. nail plate

____2. eponychium

____3. lunula

Definitions

Match the definitions in *Column I* with the words in *Column II.*

Column I	Column II
____1 the study of surface markings of the skin, especially of the palmar and plantar regions	**A** dermatoglyphics
____2 the pale arched area at the proximal portion of the nail plate; the half moon	**B** lunula
____3 fine soft hair with minute shafts and large papillae; it occurs on the forehead, ears, and flanks	**C** lanugo
____4 perspiration excreted in large quantity, or when there is much humidity in the atmosphere, so that moisture appears on the skin	**D** sensible perspiration
____5 perspiration that evaporates before it is perceived as fluid on the skin	**E** insensible perspiration

Review Questions

COMPLETION

(Circle the letter corresponding to the appropriate word or words)

1 The functions of the skin include
1. protection
2. regulation of body temperature
3. excretion of urea
4. excretion of CO_2

a. 1, 2 b. 3, 4 c. 1, 2, 3 d. all the above

2 Fingernails are totally replaced every
a. 4 weeks

b. 2 months
c. 5½ months
d. 12 months

3 Toenails are totally replaced every
a. 2 months
b. 5½ months
c. 12–18 months
d. 24–36 months

4 The first fine hair that covers the body is called
a. neelus
b. terminal
c. lanugo
d. none of the above

5 Perspiration is composed of
1. H_2O
2. CO_2 dissolved in H_2O
3. Na, Cl, K, glucose
4. urea
a. 1, 3 b. 2, 4 c. 1, 3, 4 d. all the above

INSPECTION AND PALPATION: SKIN

Behavioral Objectives

The student will be able to:

1 define in writing the terms listed under *Definitions*
2 answer in writing all *Review Questions*
3 state in writing that inspection and palpation of the skin include:
a) assessment of the skin's color, vascularity, moisture, temperature, texture, thickness, mobility, and turgor
b) description of lesions present (including color, type, configuration, morphology, and distribution over the body)
c) inspection and palpation of nails for color, shape, and lesions
d) inspection and palpation of hair for color, texture, and distribution
4 describe and record appropriately (on the check list provided) the physical findings related to inspection and palpation of the skin of three adults and three children
5 describe macule, papule, nodule, plaque, wheal, vesicle, bulla, pustule, tumor, fissure, lichenification, keloid, spider angioma, diaper rash, seborrheic dermatitis, acne
6 recognize petechiae, ecchymoses, strawberry mark, port wine stain, stork's beak mark, milia, erythema toxicum neonatorum, mongolian spots, cavernous hemangioma, and café-au-lait spots.

Learning Activities

Required

A *Read:*
Alexander and Brown, Bates

B *View:* Blue Hill Series videotapes *Physical Assessment—Integument/Lymph Nodes* and *Pediatric Examination—General Appearance, Skin, Lymph, Head, Face and Neck*

C *Examine* the skin of three adults and three children and record findings on the check list provided.

CHECK LIST

Skin: Inspection and Palpation

The following list should be filled in for each inspection and palpation required in the learning activities.

Sex______________

Age______________

General Observations	**Yes**	**No**	**Describe** (*where appropriate*)
Color (*normal*)			
brown			
cyanosis			
redness			
yellowness			
pallor			
vitiligo			
other			
Edema			
Moisture			
dryness			
sweating			
oiliness			
Temperature			
cool			
warm (*normal*)			
hot			
Texture			
rough			
smooth			
Mobility			
mobile			
stable			
flabby			
returns rapidly			
Turgor good			
Lesions			
Vascular lesions			
spider nevi			
venous star			
ecchymosis			
petechiae			
other			
Nonvascular lesions			
color			
type			
configuration (grouping)			
distribution			
morphology			

Definitions

Part I

Match the definitions in *Column I* with the correct words in *Column II*.

_____1 a small, thin plate of horny epithelium, resembling a fish scale, cast off from the skin

_____2 an outer layer or covering; a scab; a coagulation product of blood, serum, pus, or a combination of two or more of these

_____3 a scratch mark; a linear break in the skin surface, usually covered with blood or serous crusts; entire epidermis is gone, exposing the dermis

_____4 a wearing away; a state of being worn away, with loss of superficial portions of the dermis

_____5 destruction and loss of epidermis, dermis, and subcutaneous tissue

_____6 the fibrous tissue replacing normal tissues destroyed by injury or disease

_____7 a wasting of tissues, organs, or the entire body

_____8 a dark bluish or purplish coloration of the skin and mucous membrane due to deficient oxygenation of the blood in the lungs or to an abnormally great reduction in the flow of the blood through the capillaries; it appears when the reduced hemoglobin (unoxygenated) in the minute blood vessels is 5 mg or less per 100 ml

_____9 a yellowish staining of the integument, the deeper tissues, and the excretions with bile pigments

_____10 yellowish or brownish macules developing on the exposed parts of the skin, especially in persons of sandy complexion; the lesions increase in number on exposure to the sun

_____11 a strip, band, streak, or line distinguished by color, texture, depression, or elevation from the tissue in which it is found

_____12 a purplish patch caused by extravasation of blood into the skin; black and blue spot; larger than petechiae

_____13 a prominent line straight across the palms of the child's hands frequently displayed by children with Down's syndrome

_____14 broadening and thickening of ends of fingers; seen in chronic pulmonary disease, due to lack of oxygen

_____15 redness of skin

_____16 the appearance on the skin of white patches due to simple loss of pigment without other trophic changes

_____17 blackhead; a plug of sebaceous matter, capped with a blackened mass of dust and epithelial debris, filling the pilosebaceous orifice

_____18 baldness

_____19 a perceptible accumulation of excessive clear watery fluid in the tissues, which retain for a time the indentation produced by pressure

A comedo
B scar
C alopecia
D scale
E atrophy
F freckles
G pitting edema
H clubbing
I crust
J jaundice
K vitiligo
L striae
M excoriation
N cyanosis
O simian crease
P erosion
Q ecchymosis
R ulcer
S erythema

Part II

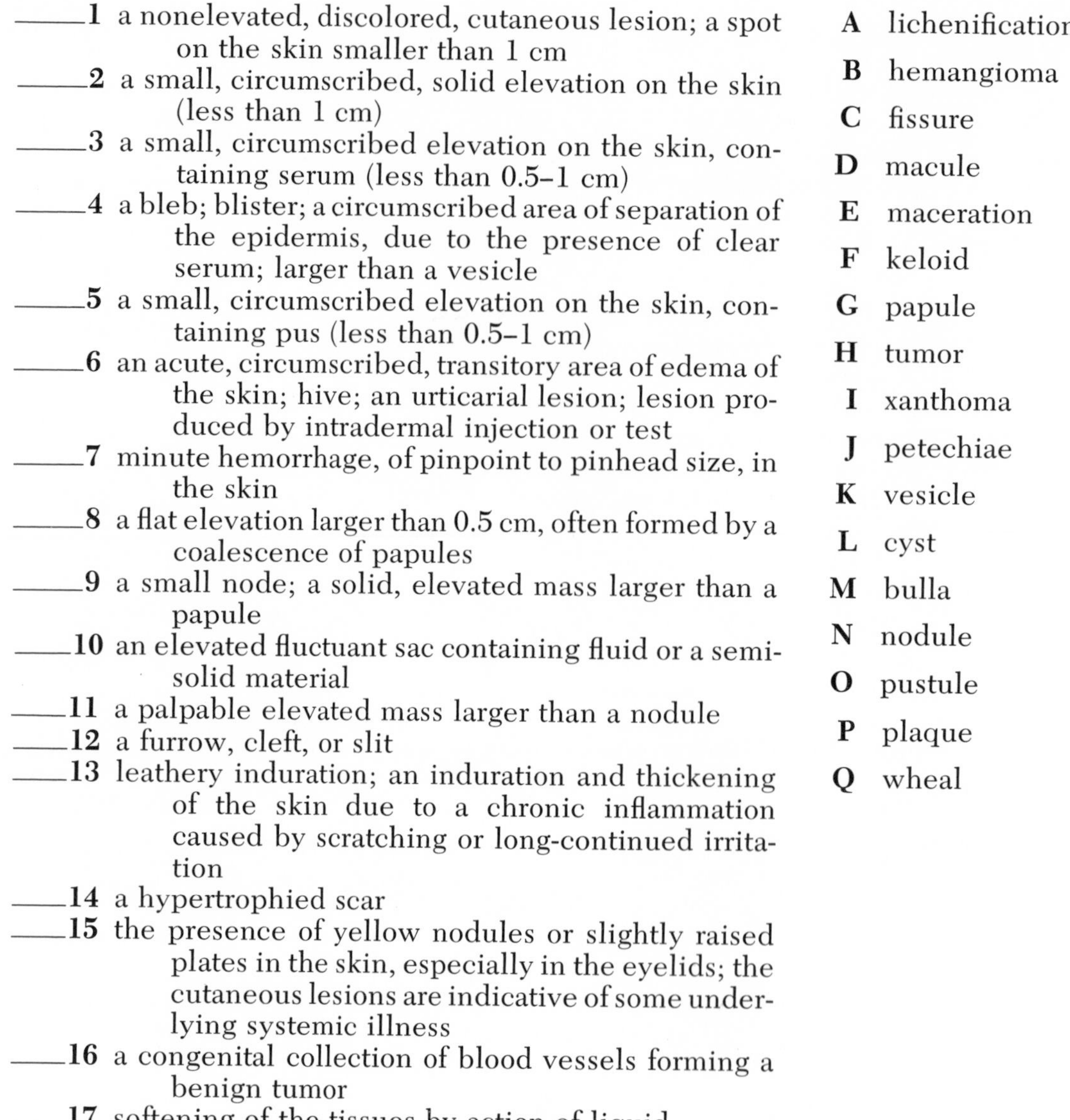

______1 a nonelevated, discolored, cutaneous lesion; a spot on the skin smaller than 1 cm

______2 a small, circumscribed, solid elevation on the skin (less than 1 cm)

______3 a small, circumscribed elevation on the skin, containing serum (less than 0.5–1 cm)

______4 a bleb; blister; a circumscribed area of separation of the epidermis, due to the presence of clear serum; larger than a vesicle

______5 a small, circumscribed elevation on the skin, containing pus (less than 0.5–1 cm)

______6 an acute, circumscribed, transitory area of edema of the skin; hive; an urticarial lesion; lesion produced by intradermal injection or test

______7 minute hemorrhage, of pinpoint to pinhead size, in the skin

______8 a flat elevation larger than 0.5 cm, often formed by a coalescence of papules

______9 a small node; a solid, elevated mass larger than a papule

______10 an elevated fluctuant sac containing fluid or a semisolid material

______11 a palpable elevated mass larger than a nodule

______12 a furrow, cleft, or slit

______13 leathery induration; an induration and thickening of the skin due to a chronic inflammation caused by scratching or long-continued irritation

______14 a hypertrophied scar

______15 the presence of yellow nodules or slightly raised plates in the skin, especially in the eyelids; the cutaneous lesions are indicative of some underlying systemic illness

______16 a congenital collection of blood vessels forming a benign tumor

______17 softening of the tissues by action of liquid

A lichenification
B hemangioma
C fissure
D macule
E maceration
F keloid
G papule
H tumor
I xanthoma
J petechiae
K vesicle
L cyst
M bulla
N nodule
O pustule
P plaque
Q wheal

Review Questions

TRUE—FALSE

Pediatric

_____1 In physiologic jaundice in newborns, jaundice appears within the first 24 hours.

_____2 Poor skin turgor is an indicator of dehydration.

_____3 Scaliness and desquamation are seldom seen in normal newborns.

_____4 Pubic hair most commonly appears at age 9–10 years.

_____5 Infants with coarctation of the aorta, below the aortic arch, may show more cyanosis in the lower extremities than in the upper extremities.

_____6 An infant with a beefy-red color over his entire body may be hypoglycemic.

_____7 Café-au-lait spots may be indicative of fibromas or neurofibromatosis.

_____8 Strawberry marks usually need excision and should be referred.

_____9 Erythema nodosum is seen in children with rheumatic fever.

_____10 Tufts of hair over the spinal and sacral region may mark a spina bifida.

_____11 Children with severe protein malnutrition often have hair tipped with a reddish rust color.

_____12 Circle the conditions that always need referral:

a) miliaria
b) seborrheic dermatitis
c) mild diaper rash
d) mild acne
e) none of the above

_____13 Mongolian spots are seen more often in the brown and black race, and have no clinical significance.

_____14 Newborns with erythema toxicum neonatorum should be isolated.

_____15 In moderate amounts, small firm mobile nodes in neck and inguinal area are generally abnormal in the child.

Adult

_____16 Diffuse or localized hyperpigmentation may be seen in Addison's disease, pregnancy, or after exposure to sunlight.

_____17 Cyanosis is usually an abnormal finding in the adult.

_____18 Canities (graying) of hair is a common finding in the adult.

Both

_____19 The normal angle of the fingernails is 160° and the shape is convex.

_____20 Very brittle dry hair may indicate hyperthyroidism.

_____21 As in jaundice, the sclera are yellow in carotinemia.

_____22 In an adult woman or preadolescent child sudden increase in facial and scalp oiliness can suggest a virilizing hormonal imbalance.

_____23 An angle of 180° between the cuticle and nail plate is a sign of early clubbing.

BASIC KNOWLEDGE: LYMPHATIC SYSTEM

Behavioral Objectives

The student will be able to:

1 answer in writing all *Review Questions*
2 label figures of superficial lymphatic system
3 state in writing the drainage patterns of the superficial lymphatic system
4 state in writing that examination of the lymphatic system includes inspection and palpation in good lighting.

Learning Activities

Required

A *Read:*
Alexander and Brown, Bates

B *Label:* Figures 2–3, 2–4, 2–5, 2–6

Figure 2–3
Lymphatic system

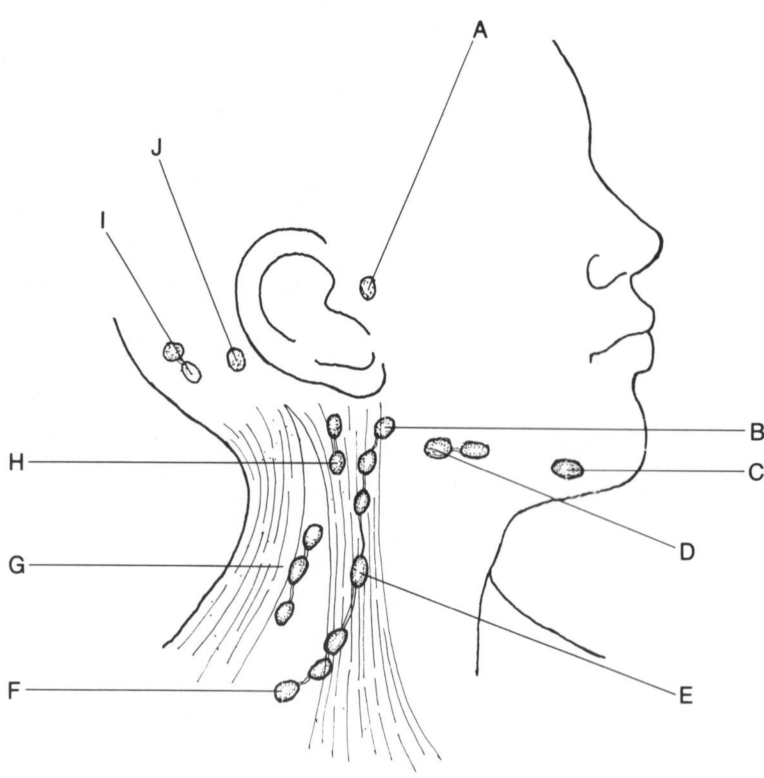

Label:

_____1. tonsillar nodes
_____2. occipital nodes
_____3. posterior cervical nodes
_____4. submaxillary nodes
_____5. supraclavicular nodes
_____6. submental nodes
_____7. posterior auricular nodes
_____8. deep cervical chain nodes
_____9. superficial cervical nodes
_____10. preauricular nodes

Figure 2–4
Lymphatic system

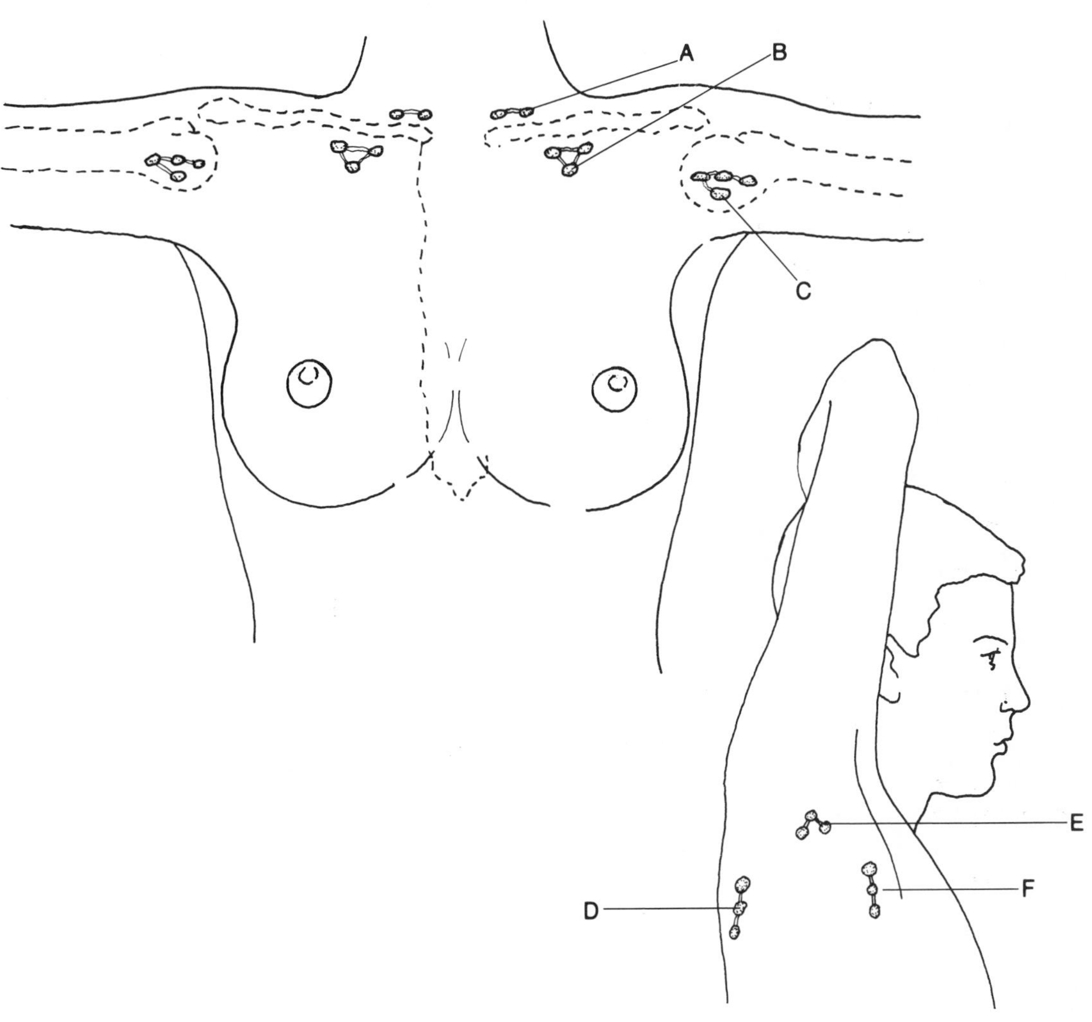

Label:

____1. infraclavicular nodes

____2. supraclavicular nodes

____3. lateral nodes

Label:

____4. central nodes

____5. subscapular nodes

____6. pectoral nodes

Figure 2–5
Lymphatic system

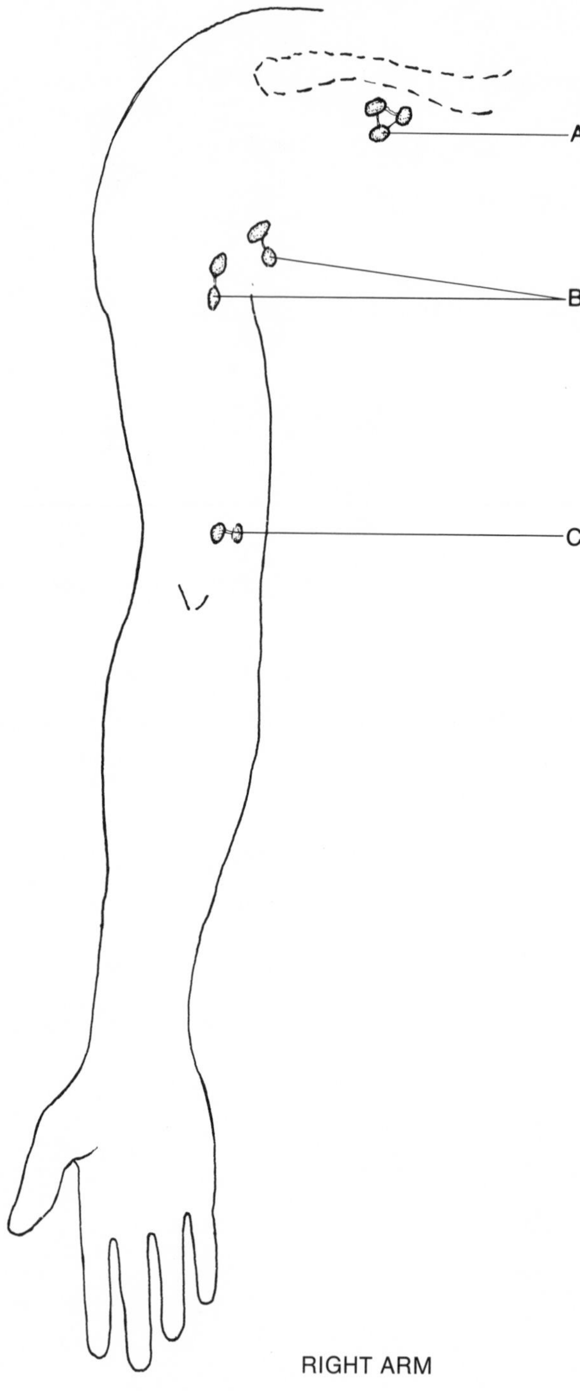

Label:

___1. infraclavicular nodes

___2. epitrochlear nodes

___3. axillary nodes

Figure 2–6
Lymphatic system

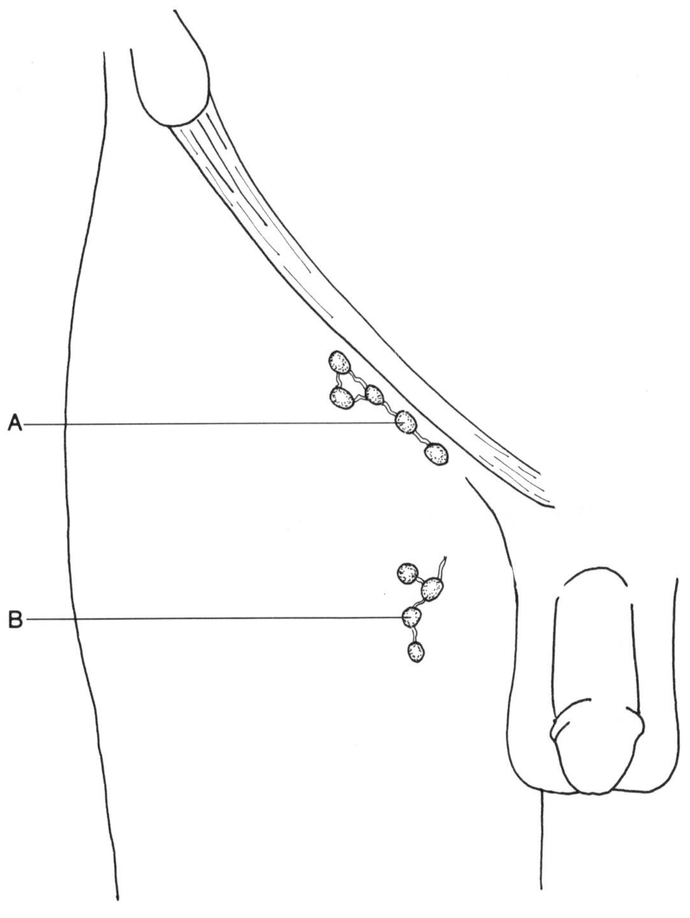

Label:

____1. vertical inguinal nodes

____2. horizontal inguinal nodes

Review Questions

MATCHING
(Match the following columns)

These organs and/or areas

_____1 tonsils
_____2 mouth
_____3 scalp
_____4 breast
_____5 posterior chest wall
_____6 upper arm
_____7 ulnar surface of forearm
_____8 external genitalia
_____9 knee

are drained by which of these lymph nodes?

a) horizontal inguinal
b) vertical inguinal
c) epitrochlear
d) lateral axillary
e) subscapular
f) supraclavicular
g) pectoral
h) submaxillar
i) cervical
j) occipital
k) supraclavicular

Multiple Choice

10 Lymph and blood mix at the:

a. jugular
b. subclavian
c. jugular and subclavian
d. none of the above

True—False

____**11** Lymph is a clear, watery fluid that flows within its own system.

INSPECTION AND PALPATION: LYMPHATIC SYSTEM

Behavioral Objectives

The student will be able to:

1 answer in writing all *Review Questions*

2 state in writing that inspection and palpation of the lymphatic system include examination of the head and neck nodes, the axillary nodes, the arm nodes, and the inguinal nodes

3 describe and record appropriately (on the check list provided) the physical findings related to inspection and palpation of the lymphatic systems of three adults and three children.

Learning Activities

Required

A *Read:*

Alexander and Brown, Bates

B *Examine* the lymphatic systems of three adults and three children and record findings on the check list provided.

CHECK LIST

Lymphatic System: Inspection and Palpation

The following list should be filled in for each inspection and palpation required in the learning activities.

Sex____________
Age____________

Location of Nodes	Yes	No	Describe (*where appropriate*) According to Characteristics Listed Below*
Head and Neck			
pre-auricular			
posterior auricular			
occipital			
tonsillar			
submaxillary			
submental			
superficial cervical			
posterior cervical chain			
deep cervical chain			
supraclavicular			
Axillary			
infraclavicular			
lateral			
central			
pectoral			
subscapular			
Epitrochlear			
Inguinal			
horizontal			
vertical			

*LYMPH NODES—CHARACTERISTICS:

Size ____ cm
Color
Temperature
Movable/fixed

Consistency
- soft
- firm
- mushy
- hard

Tender/nontender

Review Questions

MATCHING
(Match the following columns)

If the infection is:

____**1** cellulitis of ankle
____**2** cellulitis of thumb
____**3** tonsillitis
____**4** breast abscess
____**5** cellulitis of ring finger
____**6** lower abdominal abscess
____**7** scalp infection
____**8** stomatitis

You would look for lymphadenopathy in:

A cervical nodes
B submaxillary nodes
C occipital & postauricular nodes
D supraclavicular nodes
E lateral axillary nodes
F pectoral axillary nodes
G subscapular axillary nodes
H epitrochlear nodes
I horizontal inguinal nodes
J vertical inguinal nodes

TRUE—FALSE

____**1** The main concern the nurse has when examining the lymphatic system is lymphadenopathy.
____**2** If lymph nodes are enlarged, warm, and tender, it is a sign of a current infection.
____**3** Lymphadenopathy may be a sign of cancer.

Self-evaluation Key

FIGURE 2–1 (p. 5)

1. J
2. A
3. H
4. L
5. E
6. K
7. B
8. I
9. C
10. G
11. F
12. D

FIGURE 2–2 (p. 6)

1. C
2. A
3. B

DEFINITIONS—BASIC KNOWLEDGE: SKIN (p. 6)

1. A
2. B
3. C
4. D
5. E

REVIEW QUESTIONS—BASIC KNOWLEDGE: SKIN (p. 6)

1. c
2. c
3. c
4. c
5. c

DEFINITIONS—INSPECTION AND PALPATION: SKIN (pp. 9, 10)

(PART I)

1. D
2. I
3. M
4. P
5. R
6. B
7. E
8. N
9. J
10. F
11. L
12. Q
13. O
14. H
15. S
16. K
17. A
18. C
19. G

(PART II)

1. D
2. G
3. K
4. M
5. O
6. Q
7. J
8. P
9. N
10. L
11. H
12. C
13. A
14. F
15. I
16. B
17. E

REVIEW QUESTIONS—INSPECTION AND PALPATION: SKIN (p. 11)

1. F
2. T
3. F
4. F
5. T
6. T
7. T
8. F
9. F
10. T
11. T
12. e
13. T
14. F
15. F
16. T
17. T
18. T
19. T
20. F
21. F
22. T
23. T

FIGURE 2–3 (p. 12)

1. B
2. I
3. G
4. D
5. F
6. C
7. J
8. E
9. H
10. A

FIGURE 2–4 (p. 13)

1. B
2. A
3. C
4. E
5. D
6. F

FIGURE 2–5 (p. 14)

1. A
2. C
3. B

FIGURE 2–6 (p. 15)

1. B
2. A

REVIEW QUESTIONS—BASIC KNOWLEDGE: LYMPHATIC SYSTEM (pp. 15, 16)

1. I
2. H
3. J
4. G
5. E
6. D
7. C
8. A
9. B
10. C
11. T

REVIEW QUESTIONS—INSPECTION AND PALPATION: LYMPHATIC SYSTEM (p. 18)

MATCHING

1. J
2. E
3. A
4. F
5. H
6. I
7. C
8. B

TRUE—FALSE

1. T
2. T
3. T

3

head, face, and neck

TO THE STUDENT

The details on the examination of ear, eye, nose, mouth, and cardiovascular and nervous systems of the head, face, and neck will be included in other sections. Transillumination will be discussed as an additional examination method.

Recommended materials:

1 Alexander, Mary, and Brown, Marie. *Pediatric Physical Diagnosis for Nurses.* New York: McGraw-Hill Book Co., 1974.
2 Bates, Barbara. *A Guide to Physical Examination.* Philadelphia: J. B. Lippincott Co., 1974
3 Prior, John, and Silberstein, Jack. *Physical Diagnosis.* St. Louis: C. V. Mosby Co., 1973
4 "Patient Assessment—Examination of the Head and Neck." Programmed Instruction. *American Journal of Nursing* (May 1975)
5 Blue Hill Educational Systems, Inc. *Pediatric Physical Examination—General Appearance, Skin, Lymph, Head, Face and Neck* (Videotape: 48 minutes)
6 Blue Hill Educational Systems, Inc. *Physical Assessment Examinations—Head and Neck* (Videotape: 18 minutes)
7 Lippincott Visual Guide to Physical Examination. *Head and Neck* (Film/videotape: 15 minutes)
8 transilluminating flashlight
9 Ross Laboratories Transillumination Procedure (p. 33)
10 access to three adults and three children of varying ages, including an infant, who will allow you to examine their heads, faces and necks

BASIC KNOWLEDGE

Behavioral Objectives

The student will be able to:

1 answer in writing all *Review Questions*

2 label the anatomical structures of the head, face, and neck indicated in Figures 3–1, 3–2, 3–3, and 3–4
3 describe a systemic approach to performing this examination (proceeding from general to specific)
4 state in writing that examination of the head, face, and neck includes inspection and palpation.

Figure 3–1
Head

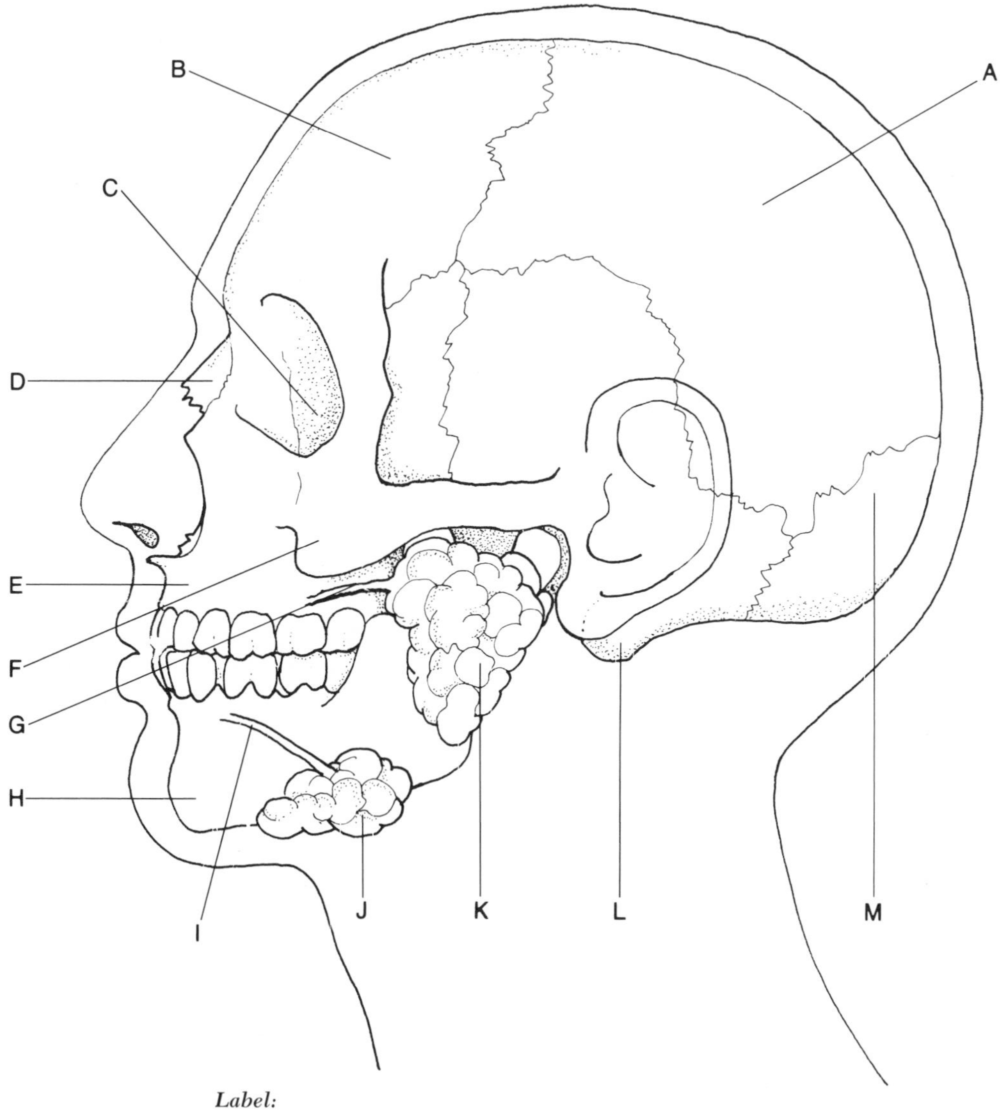

Label:

_____1. mandible
_____2. occipital bone
_____3. maxilla
_____4. parotid gland
_____5. nasal bone
_____6. mastoid process
_____7. submaxillary gland
_____8. submaxillary duct
_____9. frontal bone
_____10. zygomatic bone
_____11. parietal bone
_____12. parotid duct
_____13. orbit

Figure 3–2
Neck

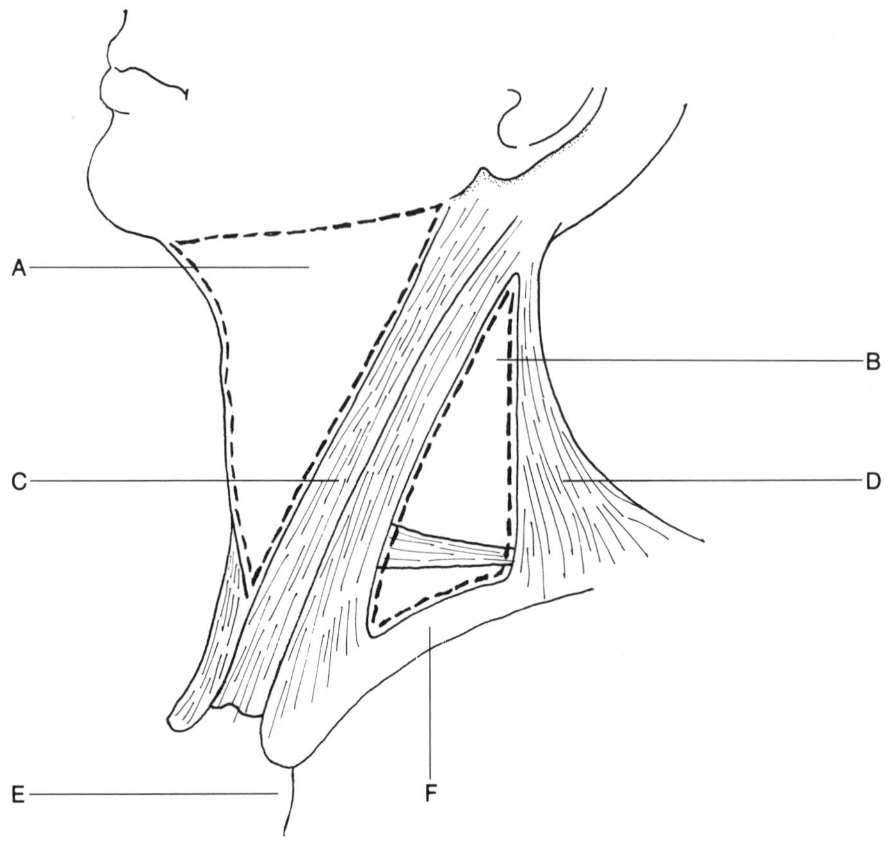

Label:

___1. sternocleidomastoid muscle	___4. clavicle
___2. manubrium of the sternum	___5. posterior triangle
___3. anterior triangle	___6. trapezium muscle

Learning Activities

I Required

A *Read:*

Alexander and Brown, Bates

AJN Programmed Instruction "Patient Assessment—Examination of the Head and Neck, Section 9, The Thyroid Gland," pp. 17–19

Ross Laboratory Transillumination Procedure (p. 33)

B *Label:* Figures 3–1, 3–2, 3–3, 3–4

C *View:* Blue Hill Series videotapes *Physical Assessment—Head and Neck* and *Pediatric Examination—General Appearance, Skin, Lymph, Head, Face and Neck*

II Optional

See listing of additional references and materials specific to head and neck in *Bibliography*.

Figure 3–3
Neck

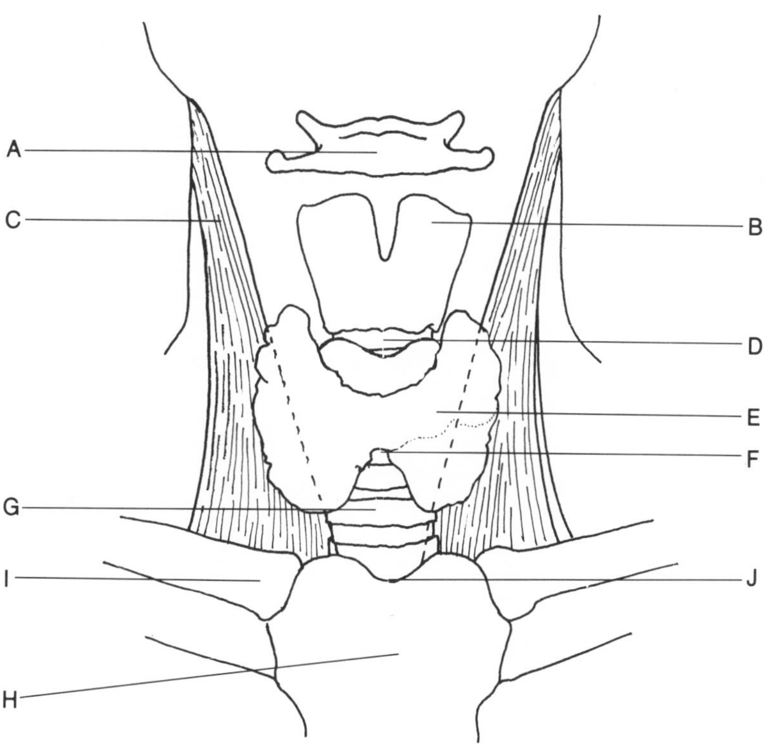

Label:

____1. sternal notch

____2. lobe of thyroid gland

____3. clavicle

____4. cricoid cartilage

____5. trachea

____6. thyroid cartilage

____7. sternocleidomastoid muscle

____8. manubrium of sternum

____9. hyoid bone

____10. isthmus of thyroid gland

Review Questions

TRUE—FALSE

____1 The sternocleidomastoid muscle turns the head to either side.
____2 The trapezius muscle turns the head and raises the shoulder.
____3 The trachea is larger in females.
____4 The thyroid secretes thyroxin, which is necessary for normal growth and development.

INSPECTION AND PALPATION

Behavioral Objectives

The student will be able to:

1 answer in writing all *Review Questions*
2 state in writing that inspection and palpation of the head, face, and neck includes:

a) measurement of head circumference in a child
b) assessment of the head for shape; symmetry; status of fontanels; hair distribution, color, and texture; movement; lymphadenopathy; and masses
c) assessment of the face for placement of features, shape, skin condition, lymphadenopathy, masses, and edema
d) assessment of the neck for shape, symmetry, movement, position of trachea, enlargement of the thyroid, lymphadenopathy, and masses.

3 palpate the thyroid correctly for enlargement and/or nodules
4 state which observations are within normal limits and which warrant further investigation

Figure 3–4
Fetal skull

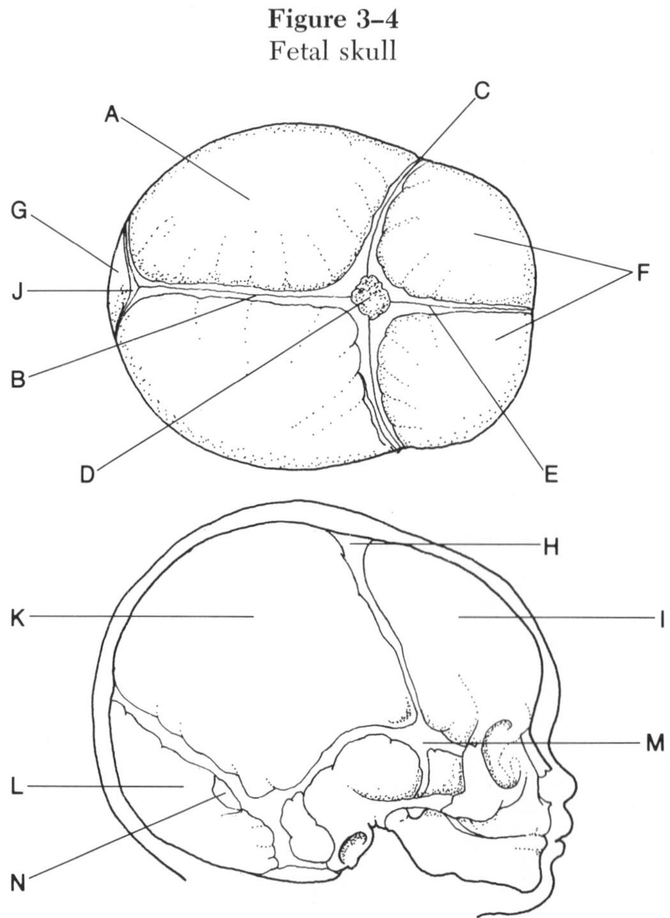

Label: **(The labels may fit more than one letter.)**

____1. lambdoidal suture	____7. sagittal suture
____2. coronal suture	____8. mastoid fontanel
____3. sphenoid fontanel	____9. posterior fontanel
____4. anterior fontanel	____10. frontal suture
____5. parietal bones	____11. occipital bone
____6. frontal bones	

5 describe and record appropriately (on the check list provided) the physical findings related to inspection and palpation of the heads, faces, and necks of three adults and three children.

Learning Activities

Required

A *Read:*

Alexander and Brown, Bates
Prior and Silberstein, pp. 63–77

B *Examine* the heads, faces, and necks of three adults and three children (including an infant under a year) and record findings on the check list provided.

CHECK LIST

Head, Face, and Neck: Inspection and Palpation

The following list should be filled in for each inspection and palpation required for the learning activities.

Sex____________________
Age____________________
Head circumference____________

	Yes	No	Describe
Head			
symmetrical			
prominent bulges			
prominent forehead			
shape of head			
normal			
long			
broad			
fontanel			
anterior: open			
closed			
size			
shape			
posterior: open			
closed			
third fontanel: size			
shape			
hair			
color even			
distribution normal			
texture			
fine			
oily			
dry			
coarse			
brittle			
amount			
thin			
thick			
alopecia			
white streak			
nits			
pediculi			

	Yes	No	Describe
scalp			
overriding sutures			
wide sutures			
dry			
flaky			
palpable nodes			
occipital			
postauricular			
movements of head			
good head control for age			
held upright			
full range of motion			
lateral			
rotation			
flexion			
extension			
temporomandibular joint			
abnormal movements			
torticollis			
bounding			
tic			
Face features			
symmetrical			
wide set eyes			
narrow set eyes			
ear pinna crosses eye occiput line			
ear attachment less than 10°			
chin decreased in size			
cheeks full			
lips full and symmetrical			
bushy eyebrows			
scant eyelashes			
brows meet in middle			
low hairline in back			
low hairline in front			
epicanthic folds			
shape			
symmetrical			

	Yes	No	Describe
moonface			
paralysis			
skin			
texture smooth			
color			
normal for race			
cyanosis			
jaundice			
hyperpigmentation			
vitiligo			
lesions			
hair present			
palpable nodes			
mandibular			
preauricular			
edema			
general			
periorbital			
Neck			
symmetrical from all angles			
skin clear			
size and shape			
short			
long			
webbing			
palpable lymph nodes			
tonsillar			
submaxillary			
superficial cervical chain			
deep cervical chain			
supraclavicular			
movement			
head rotates 90° right			
head rotates 90° left			
good muscle strength to resistance			
masses or cysts			
pulsations excessive			
trachea midline			
thyroid lobes			
palpable			

	Yes	No	Describe
enlarged			
smooth			
cricoid cartilage palpable			
thyroid cartilage palpable			
hyoid bone palpable			
thyroid isthmus palpable			
sternocleidomastoids			
symmetrical			
equal length bilaterally			
masses			

Definitions

Match the definitions in *Column I* with the correct words in *Column II*.

____1 a disorder marked by progressive enlargement of the bones of the head and face, hands and feet, and thorax, due to excessive secretion of growth hormone by the anterior lobe of the pituitary gland

____2 having a small head, denoting a skull with a capacity below 1350 cc

____3 large head; may be either congenital or acquired

____4 a condition, usually congenital, marked by an excessive accumulation of fluid in the cerebral ventricles, dilating these cavities, thinning the brain, and causing a separation of the cranial bones; there may also be an accumulation of fluid in the subarachnoid space

____5 a blood cyst of the scalp in a newborn infant, due to an effusion of blood beneath the pericranium; it does not usually cross suture lines

____6 an edematous swelling formed on the presenting portion of the scalp of an infant during birth; the effusion overlies the periosteum and consists of serum; it can cross suture lines

____7 protuberance; a circumscribed rounded swelling of the cranial vault of an infant

____8 protrusion of the eyeballs; often associated with hyperthyroidism

A caput succedaneum
B exophthalmus
C acromegaly
D bossing
E microcephalic
F cephalohematoma
G macrocephalic
H hydrocephalic

Review Questions

True—False

Pediatric

_____**1** Premature closing of the cranial suture lines may cause abnormal shape of the head and interfere with brain growth.

_____**2** Bossing in an infant is normal.

_____**3** 97% of children will have closure of the anterior fontanel between 9 and 19 months.

_____**4** Slight pulsation of the anterior fontanel is normal; great pulsations may be an indication of increased intracranial pressure.

_____**5** American Indian children have an additional horizontal suture in the occipital bone.

_____**6** For children with a white streak in their hair, hearing testing is even more important than for other children.

_____**7** Most infants have head control by two months.

_____**8** Circumoral cyanosis may be normal in the first few days of life.

_____**9** The danger of micrognathia (tiny, receding chin) to an infant is breathing difficulties due to the tongue falling backward and blocking the nasopharynx.

_____**10** The thyroid is easy to palpate in infants.

Adult

_____**11** Dyes, bleaches, and rinses not only change the color of hair but frequently make hair much coarser, drier, and more brittle.

_____**12** The thyroid is often difficult to palpate in obese adults.

Both

_____**13** Bald spots may be a sign of ringworm.

Completion
(Circle the appropriate letter)

14 When you palpate the thyroid, you should be alert to:

1) size of the isthmus
2) size of the lobes of the gland
3) its hardness
4) nodules

a) 2 b) 1, 3, 4 c) 2, 3, 4 d) all the above

15 The thyroid isthmus is located right below:

a) the thyroid lobes
b) the hyoid bone
c) the cricoid cartilage

16 Describe one method for palpation of the thyroid:

17 Describe one method for palpation of the trachea:

TRUE—FALSE

____18 100% of the adult male population is destined to have some form of alopecia.
____19 Thyrotoxicosis is often manifested by an alert, startled, and anxious appearance and by exophthalmus.
____20 Edema of the face starts in the eyelids.
____21 Excessive pulsations in the neck may be a sign of cardiac problems.
____22 Flattening of the nasal bridge and coarsening of facial features, with enlargement of the tongue, may be indicative of acromegaly.
____23 Diffuse enlargement of the thyroid is not significant.
____24 A single nodule palpated in the thyroid raises the question of malignancy.

TRANSILLUMINATION

Behavioral Objectives

The student will be able to transilluminate correctly the head of an infant.

Learning Activities

A *Read:*
Ross Laboratories Transillumination Procedure (below)

B Transilluminate and record the number of millimeters of transillumination in each of these areas of the heads of two infants:

1. R frontal
2. L frontal
3. R parietal
4. L parietal
5. occipital

State whether your findings are within normal limits.

C Define in writing the terms listed under *Definitions*.

D Answer in writing all *Review Questions*.

ROSS LABORATORIES TRANSILLUMINATION PROCEDURE*

Cranial Transillumination

Cranial transillumination is an informative procedure which can be easily done without risk to the patient. It should be included in the examination of all infants with suspected or proven neurological disorders. Hydranencephaly, hydrocephalus, porencephaly, Dandy-Walker malformation, subdural effusion, arachnoidal cyst, and cortical atrophy are among the conditions which may be suspected from transillumination. *Precise diagnosis usually demands additional studies.*

It is recommended that the procedure be used by a physician routinely at birth and at intervals during the first year of life of normal infants. Only in this way can familiarity with normal variations be gained. The method of transillumination can easily be taught to non-physicians and could be incorporated into the routine of an office or clinic much as is the measurement of height-weight.

The TRANS-DAPTER™ is a pure gum rubber attachment for a flashlight, enabling it to be used as an instrument for cranial transillumination.

Prerequisites

The TRANS-DAPTER will adapt to most standard flashlights. The flashlight should have two "D" size batteries and an opaque flange. The batteries must be fresh. There must be no leakage of light around the proximal flange of the mounted adapter. A room which can be *completely* darkened is also required—an inside office or closet is appropriate.

Technique

Allow at least three minutes in the room for dark adaptation. Position the distal flange of the TRANS-DAPTER on the baby's scalp before turning on the flashlight. Move the light slowly from front to back on comparable areas on both sides of the cranium. Note the extent of the glowing about the rim of the TRANS-DAPTER.

*Reprinted with permission of Ross Laboratories, a division of Abbott Laboratories, Columbus, Ohio 43216.

Note

The TRANS-DAPTER may be cleaned with alcohol or may be autoclaved.

References:

1. Dodge, P. R., and Porter, P. Demonstration of intracranial pathology by transillumination. Arch. Neurol. 5:594, 1961.
2. Sjogren, I., and Engsner, G. Transillumination of the skull in infants and children. Acta Paediat. Scand. 61:426, 1972.
3. Shurtleff, D. B., et al. Demonstration of intracranial pathology by transillumination. Amer. J. Dis. Child. 107:14, 1964.
4. Bray, P. E., in Neurology in Pediatrics, Chicago, Year Bk. Med., 1969, pp. 133, 143, 203, 238.
5. Gamstorp, I., in Pediatric Neurology, New York, Appleton-Century-Crofts, 1970, p. 10.

Acknowledgments:

Ross Laboratories gratefully acknowledges the cooperation and consultation of:

David W. Bailey, Captain, M.C., U.S.N.; Chief of Pediatric Service, Naval Hospital, National Naval Medical Center, Bethesda, Maryland;

Philip R. Dodge, M.D., Head, the Edward Mallinckrodt Department of Pediatrics; Professor of Pediatrics and Neurology, Washington University School of Medicine; Medical Director, St. Louis Children's Hospital; St. Louis, Missouri.

Self-Evaluation Key

FIGURE 3–1 (p. 21)

1. H
2. M
3. E
4. K
5. D
6. L
7. J
8. I
9. B
10. F
11. A
12. G
13. C

FIGURE 3–2 (p. 22)

1. C
2. E
3. A
4. F
5. B
6. D

FIGURE 3–3 (p. 23)

1. J
2. E
3. I
4. D
5. G
6. B
7. C
8. H
9. A
10. F

REVIEW QUESTIONS—BASIC KNOWLEDGE (p. 23)

1. T
2. T
3. F
4. T

FIGURE 3–4 (p. 24)

1. J
2. C
3. M
4. H, D
5. A, K
6. I, F
7. B
8. N
9. G
10. E
11. L

DEFINITIONS—INSPECTION AND PALPATION (p. 30)

1. C
2. E
3. G
4. H
5. F
6. A
7. D
8. B

REVIEW QUESTIONS—INSPECTION AND PALPATION (pp. 31, 32)

1. T
2. F
3. T
4. T
5. T
6. T
7. F
8. T
9. T
10. F
11. T
12. T
13. T
14. d
15. c
16. See Bates, pp. 46–47
17. See Bates, p. 46
18. F
19. T
20. T
21. T
22. T
23. F
24. T

4

the eye

TO THE STUDENT

The ophthalmoscopic examination is included in this section as an additional examination method.

Recommended materials:

1 Alexander, Mary, and Brown, Marie. *Pediatric Physical Diagnosis for Nurses.* New York: McGraw-Hill Book Co., 1974
2 Bates, Barbara. *A Guide to Physical Examination.* Philadelphia: J. B. Lippincott Co., 1974
3 Mechner, Francis. "Patient Assessment: Examination of the Eye, Part I." *American Journal of Nursing* 74(November 1974):2039
4 Mechner, Francis. "Patient Assessment: Examination of the Eye, Part II." *American Journal of Nursing* 75(January 1975):105
5 Blue Hill Educational Systems, Inc. *Pediatric Physical Examination—The Eye* (Videotape: 54 minutes)
6 Blue Hill Educational Systems, Inc. *Physical Assessment Examinations—Eyes* (Videotape: 45 minutes)
7 J. B. Lippincott Co. *Visual Guide to Physical Examination—Head and Neck* (Film/videotape: 14:30 minutes)
8 Colenbrander ophthalmoscopy mannequin (Hansen Ophthalmic Development Lab., P.O. Box 613, Iowa City, Iowa 52240)
9 access to three adults and three children willing to let you examine their eyes
10 access to three adults and three children willing to let you examine their eyes with an ophthalmoscope

BASIC KNOWLEDGE

Behavioral Objectives

The student will be able to:

1 answer in writing all *Review Questions*

2 identify on a live person all external anatomical structures of the eye designated in Figure 4–1
3 identify on the figure the external structures of the eye designated in Figure 4–1
4 identify the internal structures of the eye designated in Figure 4–2
5 identify the structures included in the eye musculature designated in Figure 4–3
6 identify the structures of the lacrimal system of the eye designated in Figure 4–4.

Learning Activities

I Required
  A *Read:*
    Bates, Barbara
    Alexander and Brown
    Mechner, "Patient Assessment: Examination of the Eye, Part I," pp. 2039–1 to 2039–4
  B *Label:* Figures 4–1, 4–2, 4–3, 4–4
  C *Identify* on a lab partner all external structures of the eye designated in Figure 4–1.

II Optional
    See listing of additional references and materials specific to eye in *Bibliography*.

Figure 4–1
Eye: external anatomy

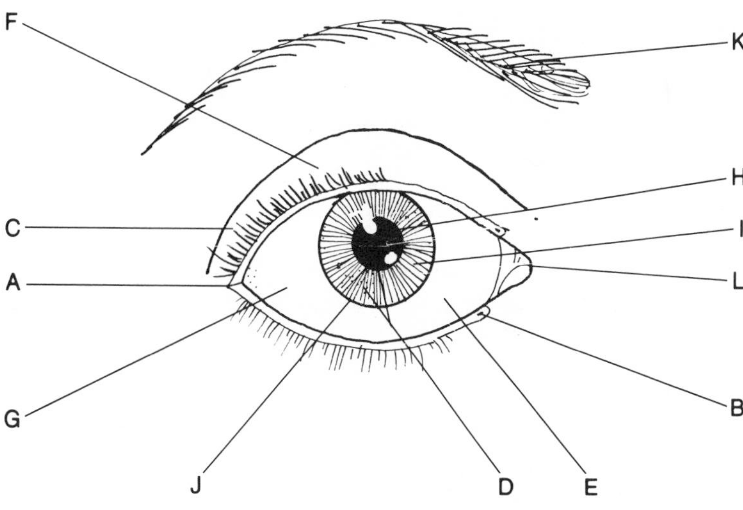

Label:

____1. sclera	____7. conjunctiva (bulbar)
____2. limbus	____8. outer canthus
____3. inner canthus	____9. pupil
____4. eyelid	____10. eyebrow
____5. lacrimal punctum	____11. cornea
____6. eyelashes	____12. iris

Figure 4–2
Eye: internal anatomy

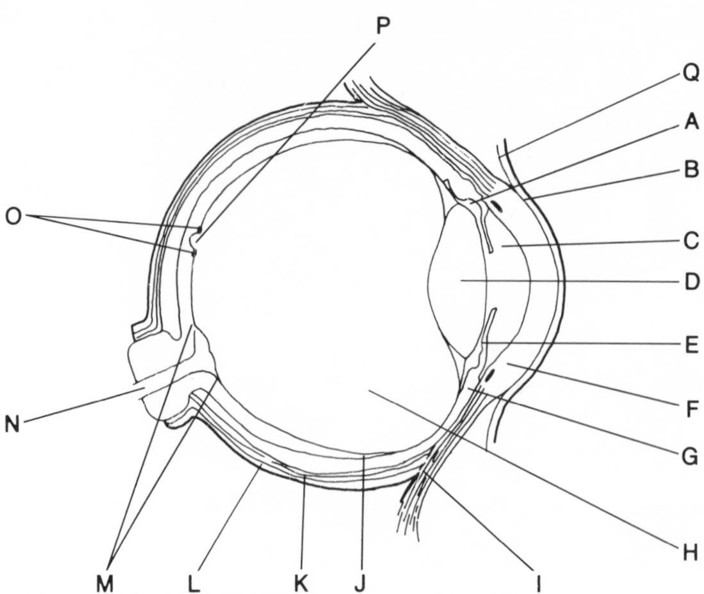

Label:

____1. iris	____7. posterior chamber	____13. choroid
____2. bulbar conjunctiva	____8. vitreous body	____14. cornea
____3. optic nerve	____9. macula	____15. medial rectus muscle
____4. retina	____10. ciliary body	____16. fovea centralis
____5. anterior chamber	____11. blind spot	____17. lens
____6. sclera	____12. corneal epithelium	

Review Questions

TRUE—FALSE

Adult

____**1** The adult eyeball is a true sphere.

Adult and Pediatric

____**2** The globe is made up of three layers.
____**3** The cornea, which covers the pupil and iris, is transparent.
____**4** The sclera, which forms the white of the eye, is opaque.
____**5** The junctional ring where the sclera joins with the cornea is called the choroid.
____**6** The retina is the innermost layer of the eye and is composed primarily of connective tissue.
____**7** The most acute vision is found in the fovea centralis.
____**8** The optic nerve transmits impulses to the posterior brain.
____**9** Normally the globe is slightly longer in length than width.
____**10** The anterior chamber is filled with vitreous humor.
____**11** The vitreous humor is a clear, viscous, gelatinous substance.
____**12** The conjunctiva is a clear, mucous membrane that covers the cornea.
____**13** The iris controls the amount of light that reaches the retina.
____**14** The palpebral conjunctiva covers the inner surface of the upper and lower lids.
____**15** The choroid is a vascular structure lying between the retina and the sclera.
____**16** The palpebral fissure is the elliptical space separating the lids when they are open.

Figure 4–3
Anatomy of the eye: musculature

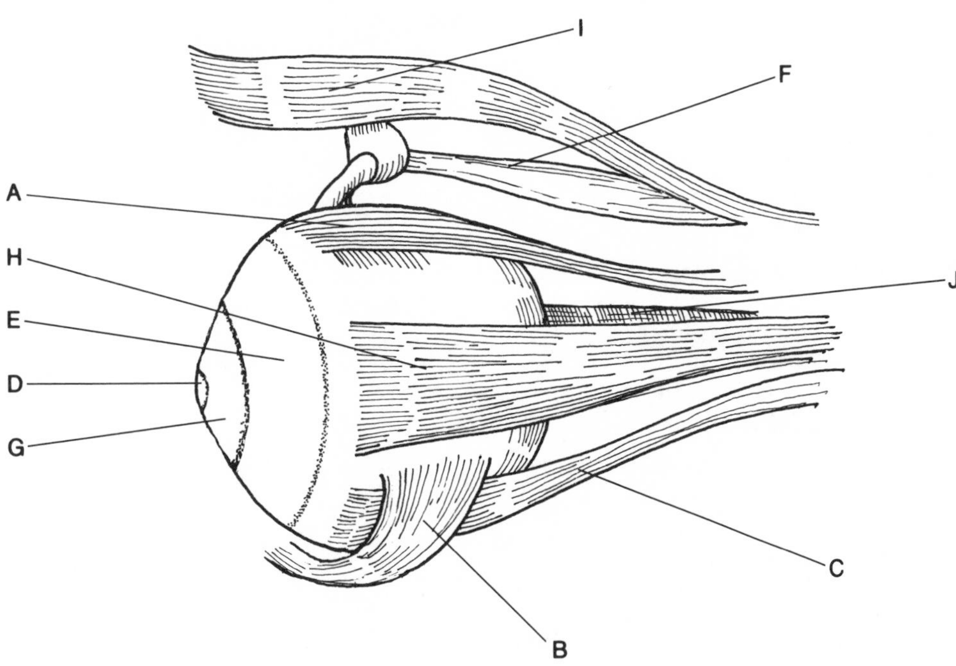

Label:

_____1. levator palpebrae superioris

_____2. pupil

_____3. rectus inferior

_____4. rectus superior

_____5. iris

_____6. rectus medialis

_____7. rectus lateralis

_____8. obliquus superior

_____9. sclera

_____10. obliquus inferior

Figure 4–4
Eye: lacrimal system

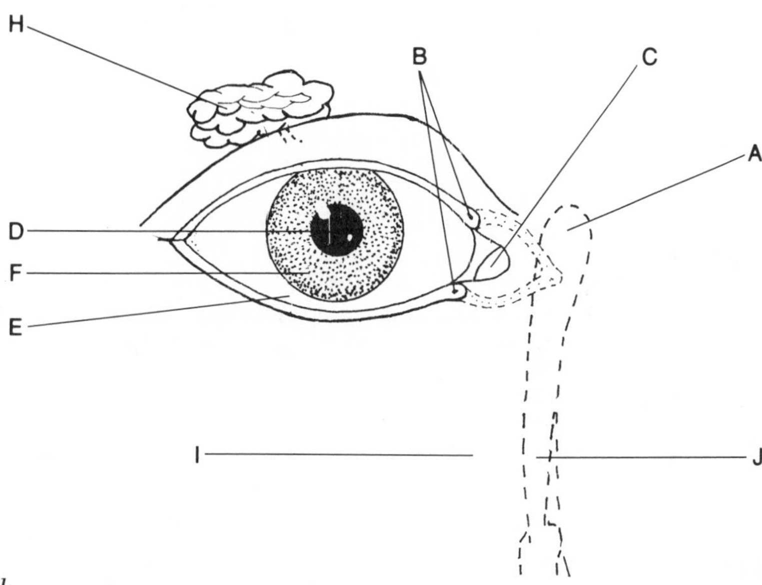

Label:

_____1. lacrimal puncta

_____2. lacrimal sac

_____3. pupil

_____4. maxillary bone

_____5. lacrimal gland

_____6. lacrimal canula

_____7. bulbar conjunctiva

_____8. nasal lacrimal duct

_____9. lacrimal duct

_____10. iris

Multiple Choice

1 The posterior chamber of the eye is filled with
   a. aqueous humor
   b. tears
   c. vitreous humor
   d. nervous tissue
   e. all the above
2 The lens is held in position by
   a. dilator muscles
   b. sphincter muscles
   c. extraocular muscles
   d. suspensory ligaments
   e. none of the above
3 The muscle that elevates the lid is the
   a. rectus superior
   b. obliquus superior
   c. rectus lateralis
   d. pupillaris superioris
   e. levator palpebrae superioris
4 The vitreous cavity of the eye is filled with
   a. aqueous humor
   b. vitreous humor
   c. lymph
   d. serum
   e. none of the above
5 Motor innervation of the levator palpebrae superioris muscle is by
   a. facial nerve
   b. trigeminal nerve
   c. oculomotor nerve
   d. abducens nerve
   e. trochlear nerve

INSPECTION

Behavioral Objectives

The student will be able to:
1 define in writing the terms listed under *Definitions*
2 answer in writing all *Review Questions*
3 label correctly the pictures in the Mechner programmed learning text, "Patient Assessment: Examination of the Eye, Part I." *AJN* (November 1974):PI 5–23
4 answer correctly the questions in the final examination concluding the Mechner programmed learning text on the eye

Learning Activities

Required
A *Read:*
   Alexander and Brown, Bates
   Mechner, pp. PI 5–24
B *View:* Blue Hill Series videotapes *Pediatric Examination—The Eye; Physical Assessment—Eyes*
C *Examine and record* on the check list provided the findings of your inspection of the eyes of three adults and three children of varying ages.

CHECK LIST
The Eye: Inspection

(To be used by the student when doing the six eye inspections required.)

Sex____________
Age____________

	RIGHT		LEFT	
	No	Yes (Describe)	No	Yes (Describe)
Lids				
ptosis				
retraction				
blepharospasm				
squinting				
setting-sun sign				
epicanthal folds				
edema				
tumors				
infections				
hordeolum				
chalazion				
furuncle				
blepharitis				
eczema				
positional faults				
ectropion				
entropion				
upward slanting				
hemangioma				
other				
Eyelashes (cilia)				
absence: partial/total				
bushy				
apigmented				
other				
Lacrimal apparatus				
lack of tearing				
excessive tearing				
infection of lacrimal sac				
other				
Palpebral conjunctiva				
color (describe)				
edema				
inflammation				

	RIGHT		LEFT	
	No	Yes (Describe)	No	Yes (Describe)
mucoid secretions				
plaques				
hemorrhage				
pterygium				
foreign body				
papilla formation				
other				
Orbit				
size (describe)				
depth (describe)				
exophthalmos				
enophthalmos				
spacing				
hypertelorism				
hypotelorism				
supraorbital ridges (describe)				
prominent				
other				
Ocular muscles				
strabismus				
Hirschberg's test				
exophoria/tropia				
esophoria/tropia				
cover test (near point)				
exophoria/tropia				
esophoria/tropia				
cover test (far point)				
exophoria/tropia				
esophoria/tropia				
diplopia				
range of motion				
upper outer				
upper inner				
lower outer				
lower inner				
lateral outer				
lateral inner				
other				
Globe				
Cornea				
enlargement				

	RIGHT		LEFT	
	No	Yes (Describe)	No	Yes (Describe)
clouding, haziness				
irritation, inflammation				
abrasion, ulceration				
dermoids				
arcus senilis				
keratoconus				
reflex				
other				
Sclera				
color (describe)				
irritation, inflamed				
abrasion, ulceration				
other				
Pupil				
irregular contour				
size				
constricted				
dilated				
symmetrical				
reaction to light—equal				
reaction to accommodation				
photophobia				
nystagmus				
other				
Iris				
color (describe)				
Brushfield's spots				
heterochromia				
coloboma				
Kayser-Fleisher ring				
hyphema				
inflammation				
prolapse				
absence (aniridia)				
other				
Lens				
dislocation				
cataract				
red reflex				

Definitions

Match the definitions in *Column I* with the correct words in *Column II*.

Part I

_____1 dimness of vision; partial loss of sight without discoverable lesion in eye structures or optic nerve
_____2 a condition in which the two pupils are not of equal size
_____3 an opaque, grayish ring at the periphery of the cornea just within the sclerocorneal junction, occurring frequently in the aged
_____4 a condition of unequal curvatures along the different meridians in one or more of the refractive surfaces
_____5 lusterless, grayish white, foamy, greasy, triangular deposits on the bulbar conjunctiva near the cornea in the area of the palpebral fissure of both eyes due to vitamin A deficiency
_____6 spasmodic winking, or contraction of the orbicularis palpebralis muscle
_____7 mottled, marbled, or speckled spots on the iris in mongolism
_____8 opacity of the crystalline lens of the eye
_____9 a small tumor of the border of the eyelid due to inflammation of a meibomian gland
_____10 edema of the ocular conjunctiva, forming a swelling around the cornea

A chalazion
B blepharospasm
C arcus senilis
D Brushfield's spots
E amblyopia
F Bitot's spots
G chemosis
H anisocoria
I cataract
J astigmatism

Part II

____11 one of a number of modified apocrine sudoriferous glands in the eyelids, with ducts that usually open into the follicles of the eyelashes
____12 a partial absence of part of the iris or deeper eye structures; when present in the iris, it causes the pupillary opening to resemble a keyhole
____13 inflammation of the conjunctiva
____14 inflammation of the lacrimal sac
____15 stricture of a lacrimal or nasal duct
____16 double vision
____17 production of inadequate amount of tears
____18 a rolling outward of the margin of an eyelid
____19 recession of the eyeball within the orbit
____20 infolding of the margin of an eyelid
____21 a fold of skin extending from the root of the nose to the inner termination of the eyebrow, overlapping the inner canthus; its presence is normal in the Oriental person
____22 a tendency of one eye to deviate inward; convergent squint
____23 a tendency of one eye to deviate outward; divergent squint
____24 protrusion of the eyeballs; often associated with hyperthyroidism
____25 a disease of the eye characterized by increased intraocular pressure due to restricted outflow of the aqueous through the aqueous veins and Schlemm's canal

A conjunctivitis
B exophthalmos
C ectropion
D ciliary glands
E esophoria
F dacryostenosis
G entropion
H diplopia
I glaucoma
J coloboma
K enophthalmos
L epicanthic folds
M dacryocystitis
N dysautonomia
O exophoria

Part III

____26 a difference in coloration between two irises
____27 a sty; an inflammation of a sebaceous gland of the eyelid
____28 farsightedness
____29 abnormally widespaced eyes
____30 hemorrhage into the anterior chamber of the eye
____31 abnormally closely spaced eyes
____32 a greenish-yellow pigmented ring encircling the cornea just within the corneoscleral margin, seen in Wilson's syndrome
____33 having abnormally large eyes
____34 jaw-winking syndrome; an increase in the width of the eyelids during chewing, sometimes with a rhythmic elevation of the upper lid when the mouth is open and ptosis when the mouth is closed
____35 inflammation of the eyelids, especially of the margins of the lids
____36 having small eyes
____37 contraction of the pupil of the eye
____38 nearsightedness
____39 rhythmical oscillation of the eyeballs, either horizontal, rotary, or vertical

A hordeolum
B myopia
C Kayser-Fleischer ring
D hypertelorism
E microphthalmia
F heterochromia
G nystagmus
H Marcus Gunn phenomenon
I hyperopia
J miosis
K hyphema
L marginal blepharitis
M hypotelorism
N macrophthalmia

Part IV

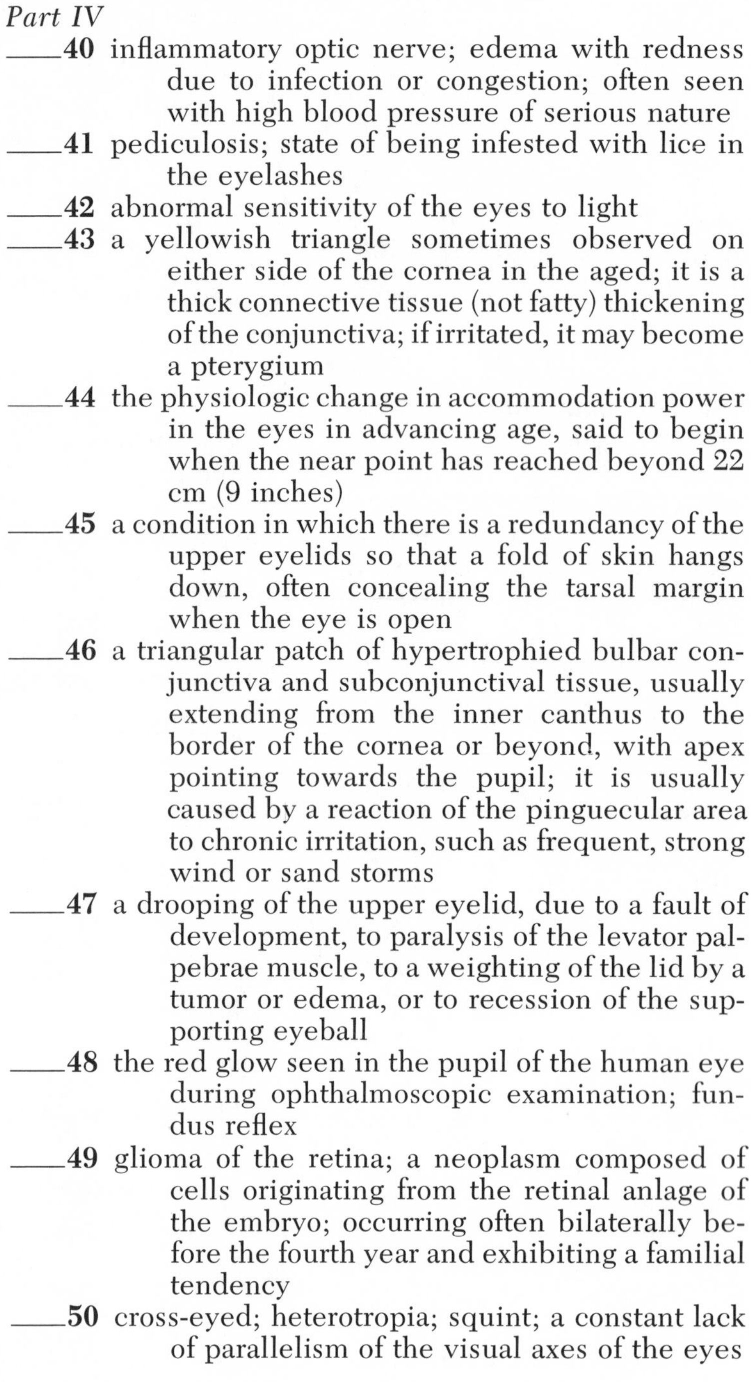

____**40** inflammatory optic nerve; edema with redness due to infection or congestion; often seen with high blood pressure of serious nature

____**41** pediculosis; state of being infested with lice in the eyelashes

____**42** abnormal sensitivity of the eyes to light

____**43** a yellowish triangle sometimes observed on either side of the cornea in the aged; it is a thick connective tissue (not fatty) thickening of the conjunctiva; if irritated, it may become a pterygium

____**44** the physiologic change in accommodation power in the eyes in advancing age, said to begin when the near point has reached beyond 22 cm (9 inches)

____**45** a condition in which there is a redundancy of the upper eyelids so that a fold of skin hangs down, often concealing the tarsal margin when the eye is open

____**46** a triangular patch of hypertrophied bulbar conjunctiva and subconjunctival tissue, usually extending from the inner canthus to the border of the cornea or beyond, with apex pointing towards the pupil; it is usually caused by a reaction of the pinguecular area to chronic irritation, such as frequent, strong wind or sand storms

____**47** a drooping of the upper eyelid, due to a fault of development, to paralysis of the levator palpebrae muscle, to a weighting of the lid by a tumor or edema, or to recession of the supporting eyeball

____**48** the red glow seen in the pupil of the human eye during ophthalmoscopic examination; fundus reflex

____**49** glioma of the retina; a neoplasm composed of cells originating from the retinal anlage of the embryo; occurring often bilaterally before the fourth year and exhibiting a familial tendency

____**50** cross-eyed; heterotropia; squint; a constant lack of parallelism of the visual axes of the eyes

A photophobia
B retinoblastoma
C epiblepharon
D papilledema
E ptosis
F presbyopia
G phthiriasis
H strabismus
I pterygium
J pinguecula
K red reflex

Review Questions

Multiple Choice

Pediatric

1 97% of epicanthal folds disappear by age
- a. 1 year
- b. 2 years
- c. 5 years
- d. 10 years
- e. 21 years

Adult and Pediatric

2 Edema of the lids might be indicative of
- a. nephritis
- b. nephrosis
- c. allergies
- d. all the above
- e. *b* and *c* only

3 Bitot's spots in the conjunctiva may be a symptom of
- a. vitamin A deficiency
- b. vitamin B deficiency
- c. hyperthyroidism
- d. glaucoma
- e. dacryostenosis

4 Brushfield's spots may be an indication of
- a. Treacher Collins syndrome
- b. Wilson's disease
- c. Down's syndrome
- d. Horner's syndrome
- e. none of the above

5 Entropion is most common in which race?
- a. Indian
- b. Oriental
- c. Caucasian
- d. Black
- e. none of the above

TRUE—FALSE

Adult

_____1 Excessive intake of vitamin A in the elderly may cause increased intracranial pressure.
_____2 Exotropia in the elderly is often self-correcting and may be ignored.
_____3 Ectropion in the elderly may be a result of loss of muscle tone.

Pediatric

_____4 An early symptom of congenital glaucoma is photophobia accompanied by tearing, blepharospasm, and corneal haziness.
_____5 Strabismus is usually insignificant in infants under age 12 months.
_____6 All cataracts can be identified only by use of the ophthalmoscope.
_____7 Ophthalmia neonatorum usually subsides without treatment.
_____8 Relative absence of tears at birth is common.
_____9 Dacryostenosis is best treated by lacrimal duct probing by 1 month of age.
_____10 Kayser-Fleischer rings often accompany juvenile diabetes.
_____11 Strabismus can often be identified by the use of the cover test and Hirschberg's test.

Both

_____12 Blepharitis is usually caused by *Staphylococcus aureus.*
_____13 Catarrhal conjunctivitis (pink eye) is always noninfectious.
_____14 Hordeolum is often caused by a staphylococcus.
_____15 Chalazion presents as a nontender mass anywhere in the tarsus of the lid.
_____16 Keratitis is an inflammation of the sclera.
_____17 Pinguecula is a malignant lesion which must be removed surgically.
_____18 Glaucoma is usually caused by blockage of the normal circulation of fluid across the surface of the eye.
_____19 Phthiriasis is usually caused by head lice.
_____20 Ptosis may result in amblyopia.
_____21 Jaundice is best detected in the sclera of the eye.

OPHTHALMOSCOPIC EXAMINATION

Behavioral Objectives

The student will be able to:

1 answer in writing all *Review Questions*

2 define in writing the terms listed under *Definitions*

3 identify on a live person the anatomical structures of the fundus designated in Figure 4–5

4 answer correctly the questions in the final quiz concluding Mechner's programmed instruction on the examination of the eye (Part II, pp. 23–24).

Learning Activities

Required

A *Read:*

Alexander and Brown

Bates

Mechner, "Patient Assessment: Examination of the Eye, Part II," pp. 105–1 to 105–22

B *View:* Blue Hill Series videotapes *Pediatric Examination—The Eye; Physical Assessment—Eyes*

C *Identify* on a lab partner all anatomical structures of the fundus listed in Figure 4–5

D *Examine* with an ophthalmoscope the eyes of three adults and three children and record findings on the check list provided.

Figure 4–5
Anatomy of the eye: fundus

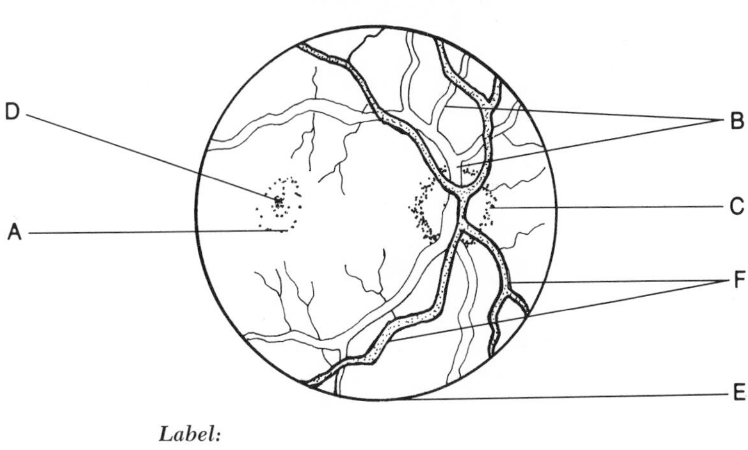

Label:

____1. **retina**	____4. **optic veins**
____2. **optic arteries**	____5. **macula**
____3. **fovea centralis**	____6. **optic disk**

CHECK LIST

Ophthalmoscopic Examination of the Eye: Inspection

(To be used by the student when doing the six ophthalmoscopic examinations required.)

Sex______________

Age______________

	RIGHT		LEFT	
Visualized:	**No**	**Yes (Describe)**	**No**	**Yes (Describe)**
Optic disk				
size				
shape				
color				
physiologic depression				
margins				
Retinal vessels				
arteries:				
size				
color				
veins:				
size				
color				
Macula				
size				
position				
Periphery				
color				
abnormalities (exudates, hemorrhages, edema)				
Media				
posterior vitreous				
anterior vitreous				
lens				

Definitions

Match the definitions in *Column I* with the correct words in *Column II*

____**1** the unit of refracting power of lenses, denoting a lens of which the principal focus is at a distance of one meter (39.3 inches)
____**2** a moderately dense opacity of the cornea
____**3** the portion of the interior of the eyeball around the posterior pole; the part exposed to view through the ophthalmoscope; eyegrounds
____**4** a degeneration of the optic disk in which it assumes a bluish gray or grayish color
____**5** a circular area of thinning of the sclera through which the fibers of the optic nerve pass
____**6** inflammatory optic nerve head; edema with redness due to injection or congestion; often seen with high blood pressure
____**7** bleeding or hemorrhage in front of the retina
____**8** a normal depression of the central part of the optic disk
____**9** dark-colored accumulation of pigment around the optic disk; this is a normal variation
____**10** a light-colored crescent at the edge of the optic disk due to a gap between the disk and the edge of the adjacent layers, revealing the underlying sclera; such a crescent is visible when the edge of the retina does not extend over the pigment concentration adjacent to the disk; this is a normal variation

A papilledema
B scleral crescent
C cataract
D physiologic cup
E diopter
F optic disk
G pigment crescent
H ocular fundus
I preretinal hemorrhage
J optic atrophy

Review Questions

True—False

_____1 The proper way to position the ophthalmoscope when examining the patient's eye is to hold the instrument in the left hand while the examiner looks through his left eye.
_____2 The fundus refers only to the optic disk and macula.
_____3 The diameter of the macula and that of the disk are about the same.
_____4 Pigmentation of the fundus varies with skin tones.
_____5 The diameter of the physiologic cup is normally less than about half the diameter of the disk.
_____6 An increase in the depth and width of the physiologic cup normally appears with aging.
_____7 Swelling of the optic nerve head is usually an indication of increased intracranial pressure.
_____8 Pallor of the entire disk is usually indicative of anemia.
_____9 Initially, the lens of the ophthalmoscope should be set at −8 while approaching the patient from a distance of about 12 inches.
_____10 In a darkened room, the red reflex can be noted in the patient's eye at a distance of 12 inches, when the ophthalmoscope is correctly focused.

Multiple Choice

1 While examining the blood vessels in the normal fundus, one notes that
  a. veins are darker in color and wider in diameter than arteries
  b. veins are darker in color and narrower in diameter than arteries
  c. veins are lighter in color and wider in diameter than arteries
  d. veins are lighter in color and narrower in diameter than arteries

2 Which of the following is an abnormal ophthalmoscopic finding of the disk?
  a. scleral crescent
  b. pigment crescent
  c. myelinated nerve fibers
  d. elongation
  e. swelling of the margins

3 The fovea normally may be visualized as the
  a. small, darker area near the center of the macula
  b. small, lighter area near the center of the macula
  c. small, darker area near the center of the disk
  d. small, lighter area near the center of the disk

4 Which of the following is a normal ophthalmoscopic finding of the macula?
  a. exudates
  b. hemorrhages
  c. scars
  d. uneven distribution of pigment
  e. avascular appearance

5 A gray or silvery area elevated above the retinal level most likely indicates
  a. diabetic retinopathy
  b. cholesterol deposit
  c. detached retina
  d. glaucoma
  e. papilledema

6 Which of the following diseases may affect the retina?
- a. diabetes
- b. hypertension
- c. leukemia
- d. arteriosclerosis
- e. all the above

Self-Evaluation Key

FIGURE 4–1 (p. 37)

1. G
2. J
3. L
4. F
5. B
6. C
7. E
8. A
9. H
10. K
11. D
12. I

FIGURE 4–2 (p. 38)

1. E
2. Q
3. N
4. J
5. C
6. L
7. A
8. H
9. O
10. G
11. M
12. B
13. K
14. F
15. I
16. P
17. D

FIGURE 4–3 (p. 39)

1. I
2. D
3. C
4. A
5. G
6. J
7. H
8. F
9. E
10. B

FIGURE 4–4 (p. 39)

1. B
2. A
3. D
4. I
5. H
6. C
7. E
8. J
9. G
10. F

REVIEW QUESTIONS—BASIC KNOWLEDGE

TRUE—FALSE (p. 38)

1. F
2. T
3. T
4. T
5. F
6. F
7. T
8. T
9. T
10. F
11. T
12. F
13. T
14. T
15. T
16. T

MULTIPLE CHOICE (p. 40)

1. a
2. d
3. e
4. b
5. c

DEFINITIONS—INSPECTION

PART I (p. 44)

1. E
2. H
3. C
4. J
5. F
6. B
7. D
8. I
9. A
10. G

PART II (p. 45)

11. D
12. J
13. A
14. M
15. F
16. H
17. N
18. C
19. K
20. G
21. L
22. E
23. O
24. B
25. I

PART III (p. 45)

26. F
27. A
28. I
29. D
30. K
31. M
32. C
33. N
34. H
35. L
36. E
37. J
38. B
39. G

PART IV (p. 46)

40. D
41. G
42. A
43. J
44. F
45. C
46. I
47. E
48. K
49. B
50. H

REVIEW QUESTIONS—INSPECTION (pp. 47, 48)

MULTIPLE CHOICE (p. 47)

1. d
2. d
3. a
4. c
5. e

TRUE—FALSE (p. 48)

1. T
2. F
3. T
4. T
5. F
6. F
7. F
8. T
9. F
10. F
11. T
12. T
13. F
14. T
15. T
16. F
17. F
18. F
19. T
20. T
21. T

FIGURE 4–5 (p. 49)

1. E
2. B
3. D
4. F
5. A
6. C

DEFINITIONS—OPHTHALMOSCOPIC EXAM (p. 51)

1. E
2. C
3. H
4. J
5. F
6. A
7. I
8. D
9. G
10. B

REVIEW QUESTIONS—OPHTHALMOSCOPIC EXAM (pp. 52, 53)

TRUE—FALSE (p. 52)

1. T
2. F
3. T
4. T
5. T
6. F
7. T
8. F
9. F
10. T

MULTIPLE CHOICE (pp. 52, 53)

1. a
2. e
3. a
4. e
5. c
6. e

5

the ear

TO THE STUDENT

Recommended materials:

1 Alexander, Mary, and Brown, Marie. *Pediatric Diagnosis for Nurses.* New York: McGraw-Hill Book Co., 1974
2 Bates, Barbara. *A Guide to Physical Examination.* Philadelphia: J. B. Lippincott Co., 1974
3 "Patient Assessment—Examination of the Ear." Programmed Instruction. *American Journal of Nursing* 75, 3 (March 1975)
4 Blue Hill Educational Systems, Inc. *Pediatric Physical Examination—Ear, Nose, Mouth and Throat* (Videotape: 53 minutes)
5 Blue Hill Educational Systems, Inc. *Physical Assessment Examinations—Ear, Nose, Throat and Mouth* (Videotape: 19 minutes)
6 J. B. Lippincott Co. *Visual Guide to Physical Examination—Head and Neck* (Film/videotape: 14:30 minutes)
7 access to three individuals willing to let you examine their ears
8 an otoscope

BASIC KNOWLEDGE, INSPECTION, AND PALPATION

Behavioral Objectives

The student will be able to:

1 answer in writing all *Review Questions*
2 answer in writing questions 1–15 in the *American Journal of Nursing* Programmed Text "Physical Examination of the Ear"
3 label the following structures on Figure 5–1: concha, helix, antihelix, tragus, antitragus, mastoid process, lobe
4 label on Figure 5–2 the following structures: handle, batteries, head, speculum, pneumonic device, lens, neck, spigot

5 label on Figure 5–3 the following structures: concha, semicircular canals, oval window, stapes, incus, malleus, eustachian tube, vestibule, external meatus, auricle, tympanic membrane, cochlea
6 label on Figure 5–4 the following commonly seen structures: tympanic membrane, annulus, pars flaccida, pars tensa, long process, short process, umbo, anterior folds, posterior folds; and also the following less commonly seen structures: chordae tympanii, shadow of the incus, (or crus of the incus), round window, and entrance of the eustachian tube
7 examine a person's ear and record findings according to the check list provided.

Learning Activities

I Required
  A *Read:*
    AJN Programmed Instruction "Patient Assessment: Examination of the Ear," pp. 1–3
    Alexander and Brown, Bates
  B *Study and label:*
    1 Figure 5–1 (according to Bates)
    2 Figure 5–2 (according to Alexander and Brown)
    3 Figure 5–3 (according to *American Journal of Nursing*, p. 2)
    4 Figure 5–4 (according to the description of landmarks on the tympanic membrane on p. 59)

Figure 5–1
External ear: landmarks

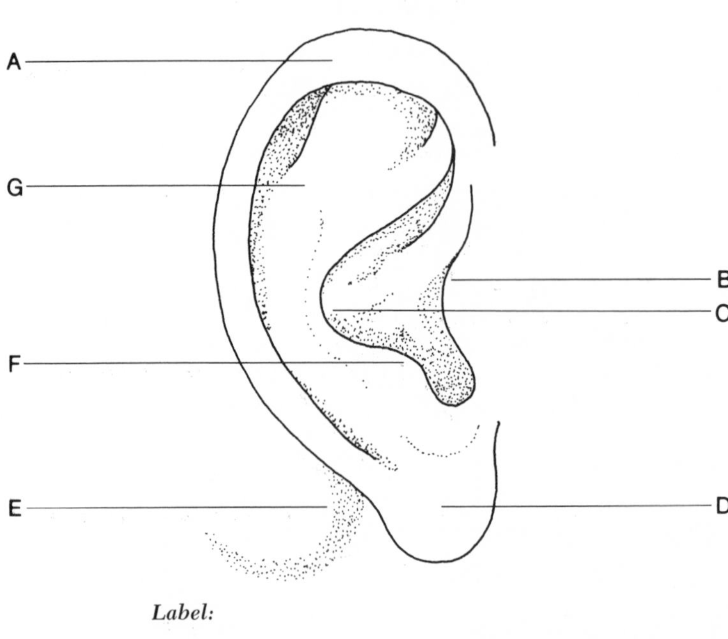

Label:

____1. lobe
____2. helix
____3. tragus
____4. mastoid process
____5. antihelix
____6. concha
____7. antitragus

C Using the otoscope, examine the ears of three individuals; include the following:

a) an evaluation of the auricle (by inspection and palpation)
b) an evaluation of the mastoid process (by inspection and palpation)
c) evaluation of the external canal
d) evaluation of the tympanic membrane, including location of the light reflex, umbo, long process, short process, annulus, pars tensa, pars flaccida, anterior and posterior malleolar folds and, if present, the crus of the incus, chordae tympanii, round window and entrance of the eustachian tube.

II Optional

See listing of additional references and materials specific to ear in *Bibliography*.

Figure 5–2
Otoscope

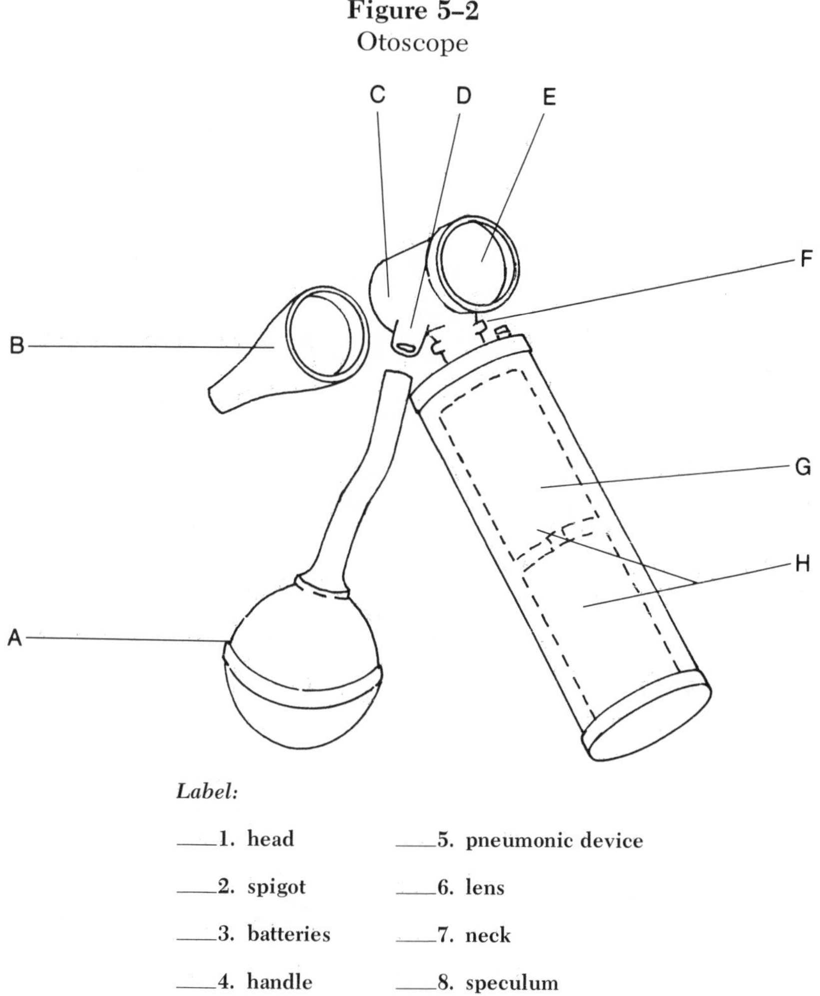

Label:

____1. **head**
____2. **spigot**
____3. **batteries**
____4. **handle**
____5. **pneumonic device**
____6. **lens**
____7. **neck**
____8. **speculum**

Figure 5–3
Ear: cross section

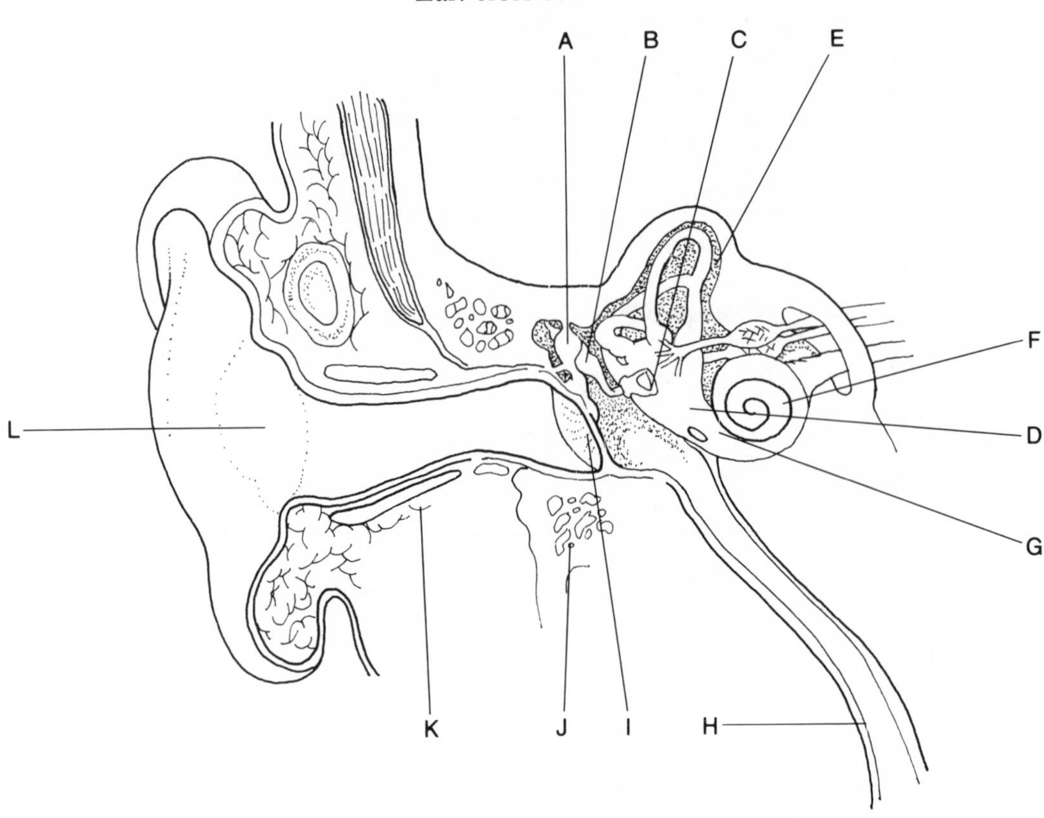

Label:

_____1. cartilaginous walls of the meatus

_____2. semicircular canals

_____3. oval window

_____4. cochlea

_____5. stapes

_____6. malleus

_____7. incus

_____8. eustachian tube

_____9. vestibule

_____10. bony walls of the meatus

_____11. auricle

_____12. tympanic membrane

Figure 5–4
Ear: tympanic membrane, landmarks

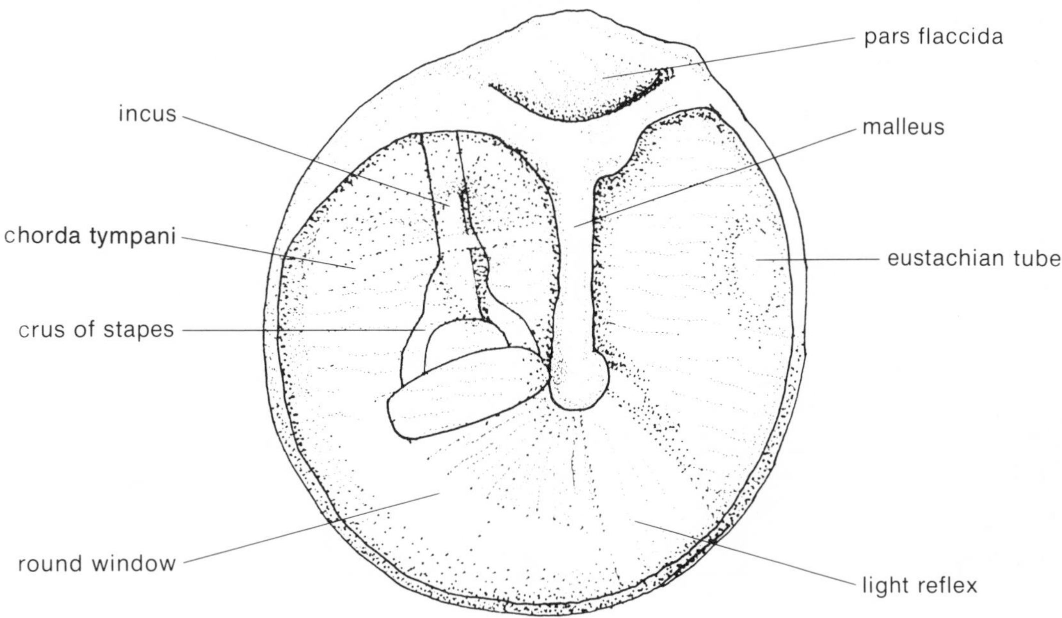

Right Ear

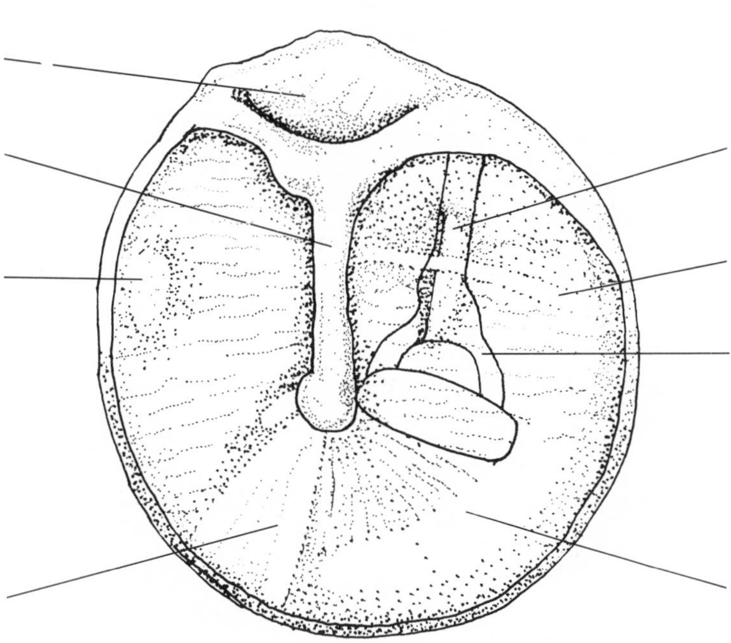

Left Ear

The books you have read for your required reading have shown you how to identify the landmarks commonly seen on the tympanic membrane. You should attempt to find these landmarks on every ear you examine. On many ears, however, you will see other landmarks which you may not recognize. The above labeled diagram shows some of these less commonly seen landmarks. It is important for you to be aware of these landmarks also and to be able to recognize them. It will help you to avoid considering them abnormal when they are seen. Fill in the lower diagram according to the completed one at the top, learning the appropriate landmarks while you do so.

CHECK LIST
Ear Examinations

Variable	Present	Not Present	Describe
Mastoid process			
tenderness			
erythema			
swelling			
other			
Auricle (pinna)			
concha			
helix			
antihelix			
tragus			
antitragus			
lobe			
darwinian tubercle			
placement			
Does it touch eye-occiput line?			
Does it deviate more than 10° from a line perpendicular to the eye-occiput line?			
External canal			
scaling			
redness			
swelling			
polyps			
tenderness			
Tympanic membrane			
annulus			
pars flaccida			
pars tensa			
long process			
short process			
umbo			
anterior fold			
posterior fold			
chordae tympanii			
crus of the incus			
round window			
entrance to eustachian tube			
holes			
bubbles			
fluid level			
retraction			
mobility			
bulging			
redness			

Review Questions

COMPLETION

(*Underline* or *write in* the word(s) or phrase(s) that complete(s) the statement.)

Pediatric

1 The tip of the pinna should cross the (eye-occiput; nose-occiput; suture) line.

2 The tympanic membrane of an infant is at an almost (vertical; horizontal) angle to the examiner's eye (when an otoscope is used).

3 If a line is drawn at right angles to the eye-occiput line, the normal ear will deviate not more than ______ degrees posteriorly.

4 The nurse should explain to mothers of small children that (it is very important to remove the cerumen at least every other day; it is not necessary to remove the ear cerumen any more than every week, but it should be done at that time carefully with a cotton tipped swab; the child's ears should be cleaned with a washcloth, but nothing should be inserted into the ear).

Adult and Pediatric

5 The patient's head should be (tilted away from the examiner; tilted toward the examiner; straight; tilted toward the ceiling; tilted toward the floor) when his ears are being examined.

6 An otoscope light that gradually turns yellow probably indicates that a new (bulb; set of batteries) is needed.

7 The normal color of the tympanic membrane is (yellow; gray; amber; blue).

8 One of the more likely spots to find perforations in the eardrum is the (annulus; long process; umbo; light reflex).

9 When you are looking at an eardrum, the quadrant farthest from you is the (posterosuperior; anteroinferior; posteroinferior; anterosuperior) quadrant.

10 If there is any possibility of a perforation in the tympanic membrane, the examiner should be careful *not to remove* cerumen with (the irrigation method; the cotton-tipped applicator; the curette).

11 Jerky movement of the tympanic membrane indicates (a normal resistance; an increased resistance; a decreased resistance) of the middle ear.

12 If the water used in irrigating the ear is too cold or too warm, the patient may experience (dizziness; stomach cramps; loss of vision).

SELECTION

(Place check marks beside the correct answers)

13 Which of the following findings warrant referral for treatment?

______1 a retracted tympanic membrane
______2 a bulging tympanic membrane
______3 a visible long process
______4 a visible air bubble
______5 a visible fluid line
______6 a visible pars flaccida
______7 a visible umbo
______8 a visible perforation
______9 a visible annulus
______10 a visible stapes
______11 a gray tympanic membrane
______12 a red tympanic membrane
______13 a tender mastoid process
______14 a mastoid process located behind the ear
______15 an auricle which extends above the eye-occiput line
______16 an auricle with a visible darwinian tubercle

Self-Evaluation Key

FIGURE 5–1 (p. 56)

1. D
2. A
3. B
4. E
5. G
6. C
7. F

FIGURE 5–2 (p. 57)

1. C
2. D
3. H
4. G
5. A
6. E
7. F
8. B

FIGURE 5–3 (p. 58)

1. K
2. E
3. D
4. F
5. C
6. A
7. B
8. H
9. G
10. J
11. L
12. I

REVIEW QUESTIONS (p. 61)

1. eye-occiput
2. horizontal
3. 10
4. child's ears should be cleaned with a washcloth, but nothing should be inserted into the ears
5. tilted away from the examiner and toward the ceiling
6. set of batteries
7. gray
8. annulus
9. anteroinferior
10. the irrigation method
11. an increased resistance
12. dizziness
13. 1,2,4,5,8,12,13

6

nose, mouth, and throat

TO THE STUDENT

This section will include the examination of the nose, nasal passages, paranasal sinuses, mouth, dentition, and throat.

Recommended materials:

1 Alexander, Mary, and Brown, Marie. *Pediatric Diagnosis for Nurses.* New York: McGraw-Hill Book Co., 1974
2 Bates, Barbara. *A Guide to Physical Examination.* Philadelphia: J. B. Lippincott Co., 1974
3 Mechner, Francis. "Patient Assessment: Examination of the Head and Neck." *American Journal of Nursing* (May 1975):frames 2.0–7.30; pp. 3–8, 11–15
4 Blue Hill Educational Systems, Inc. *Pediatric Physical Examination—Ear, Nose, Mouth and Throat* (Videotape: 53 minutes)
5 Blue Hill Educational Systems, Inc. *Physical Assessment Examinations—Ear, Nose, Throat and Mouth* (Videotape: 19 minutes)
6 J. B. Lippincott Co. *Visual Guide to Physical Examination—Head and Neck* (Film/videotape: 14:30 minutes)
7 disposable examining mirror
8 flashlight with mirror adaptor
9 penlight and tongue blades
10 otoscope and stethoscope
11 access to three adults and three children who will allow you to examine their noses, mouths, and throats

PHYSICAL EXAMINATION: NOSE

Behavioral Objectives

The student will be able to:

1 answer in writing all *Review Questions*
2 define in writing the terms listed under *Definitions*

3 identify and label the following anatomical structures on Figure 6–1: inferior turbinate, inferior meatus, middle turbinate, middle meatus, superior turbinate, superior meatus, vestibule
4 demonstrate the proper technique for examining the nose (including palpation, inspection, and auscultation)
5 accurately record the findings of a nasal examination related to: external configuration; patency, color, and consistency of nasal mucosa; structures visualized; and status of the paranasal sinuses
6 identify and label the four paranasal sinuses on Figures 6–2 and 6–3 (lateral view)
7 demonstrate the proper technique for palpation, percussion, and transillumination of the maxillary and frontal sinuses
8 answer questions from frames 2.0–4.4 and pages 3–8 in *AJN* (May 1975) programmed instruction.

Learning Activities

I Required
- A *Read:* Alexander and Brown, Bates
- B *View:* Blue Hill Series videotapes *Pediatric Examination—Ear, Nose, Mouth and Throat; Physical Assessment—Ear, Nose, Throat and Mouth*
- C *Label:* Figures 6–1, 6–2, and 6–3
- D *Complete:* list of definitions
- E *Complete:* programmed learning in *American Journal of Nursing* (May 1975):frames 2.0–4.4; pp. 3–8
- F *Examine* the noses of three children and three adults and record the findings on the check list provided. (Be sure to include transillumination data.)

Figure 6–1
Nose

A
B
C
D
E
F
G

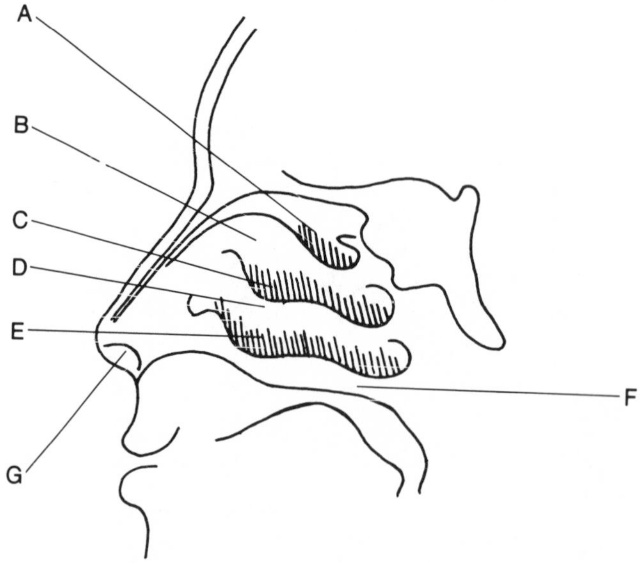

Label:

____1. **inferior turbinate** ____5. **superior turbinate**

____2. **inferior meatus** ____6. **superior meatus**

____3. **middle turbinate** ____7. **vestibule**

____4. **middle meatus**

II Optional

See listing of additional references and materials specific to nose, mouth, and throat in *Bibliography*.

Definitions

Match the definitions in *Column I* with the correct words in *Column II*.

____**1** nosebleed
____**2** nostril; the anterior opening of the nasal fossa
____**3** the upper portion of the pharynx, above the level of the palate
____**4** an inspiratory widening (by using nasal muscles) of the nostrils, often seen in patients with respiratory distress
____**5** dividing wall between the two nasal cavities, formed posteriorly of bone, anteriorly of cartilage
____**6** lower margin of the nasal septum
____**7** congenital failure of one or both sides of the nose to communicate with the pharynx

A columella
B nasal flaring
C choanal atresia
D epistaxis
E nasopharynx
F septum
G nares

Figure 6–2
Paranasal sinuses

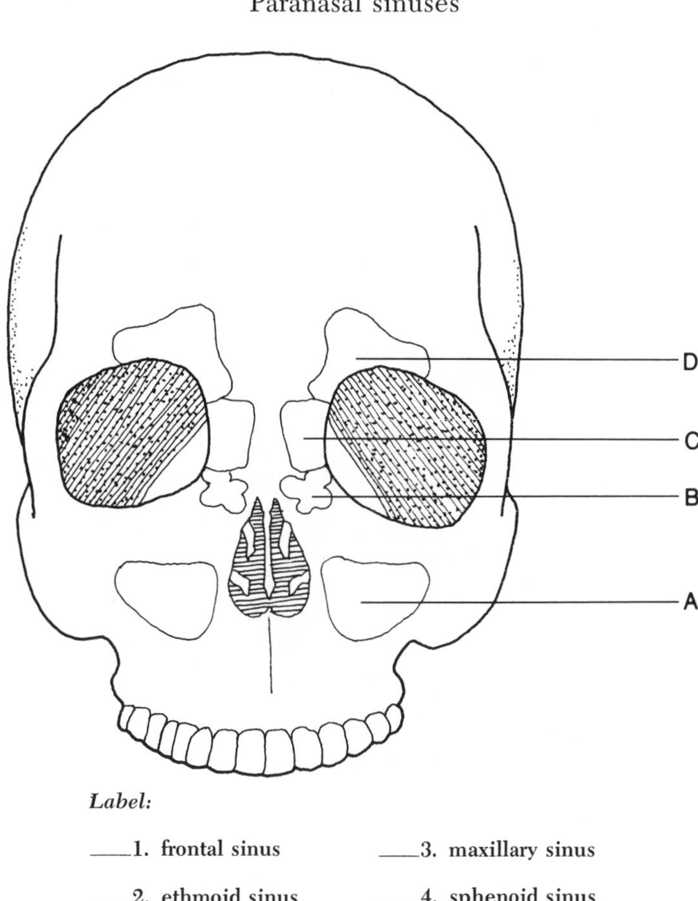

Label:

____**1. frontal sinus**
____**2. ethmoid sinus**
____**3. maxillary sinus**
____**4. sphenoid sinus**

Figure 6–3
Paranasal sinuses

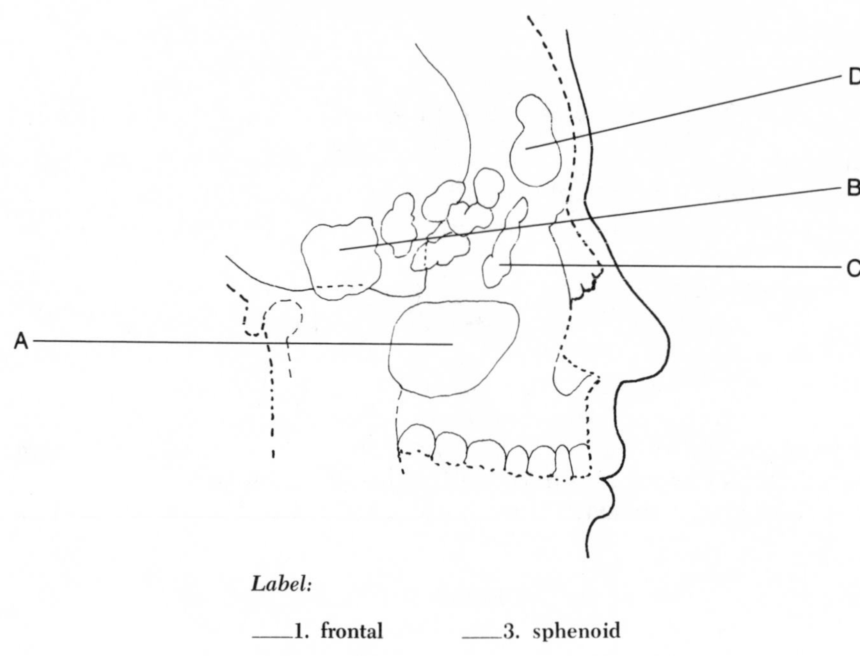

Label:

____1. frontal
____2. ethmoid
____3. sphenoid
____4. maxillary

CHECK LIST
Physical Examination: Nose

	Yes	No	Describe (*where appropriate*)
Nose normal external configuration			
patency			
nasal mucosa			
polyps			
swelling			
bleeding			
discharge			
describe color and consistency			
septum			
midline			
deviated			
Sinuses maxillary			
tender			
transilluminates			
frontal			
tender			
transilluminates			

Review Questions

Multiple Choice
(Mark the correct answer or answers)

Adult and Pediatric

1 Abnormalities in the shape of the nose are of medical concern because
- a) they may be the cause of an obstruction to the smooth flow of air
- b) they may present the patient with a cosmetic problem
- c) they can be a sign of diabetes
- d) *a* and *c*
- e) *a* and *b*

2 The nasal mucus contains enzymes that
- a) generate antibodies to combat allergies
- b) destroy bacteria
- c) digest dust and soot
- d) mobilize cilia

3 One sign by which allergies may be distinguished from the common cold is that in allergies
- a) the nasal mucosa is red, inflamed, and swollen
- b) the nasal mucosa is comparatively pale
- c) the discharge is clear and watery at the beginning
- d) the presence of nasal congestion is prominent

4 Long-term inflammation and infection of the nasal mucosa may
- a) render the mucous membrane of the nose ineffective
- b) lead to allergies
- c) result in increasing amounts of mucous secretion
- d) cause edema of the mucous membrane

5 The fact that the condition of nasal discharge includes some slight fever
- a) increases the likelihood that it is an allergy
- b) decreases the likelihood that it is an allergy
- c) has no bearing
- d) is a common finding

6 The two sets of sinuses most commonly involved in sinus infections are the
- a) frontal sinuses and maxillary sinuses
- b) maxillary sinuses and ethmoid sinuses
- c) ethmoid sinuses and sphenoid sinuses
- d) sphenoid sinuses and frontal sinuses

7 Anosmia could be the result of
- a) destruction of the nasal mucosa
- b) a neurological problem
- c) obstruction of the nasal passageways
- d) all the above
- e) *a* and *c* only

8 When faced with a patient who has a nosebleed, you should
- a) pinch the tip of the nose to stop the bleeding
- b) observe the patient carefully to see whether he is swallowing blood
- c) pinch the bridge of the nose to stop the bleeding
- d) *a* and *b*
- e) *b* and *c*

9 Epistaxis can be caused by
- a) dryness
- b) nose picking
- c) foreign objects
- d) all the above

10 The function of the turbinates is to
- a) support the cartilaginous septum
- b) trap foreign objects
- c) temper the air
- d) divide the nasal cavities

11 What proportion of the nose is bone?
- a) ¼
- b) ½
- c) ⅔
- d) ⅓

12 Which of the sinuses are readily accessible to clinical examination?
- a) sphenoid
- b) frontal
- c) maxillary
- d) all the above
- e) *b* and *c*

13 A pale, boggy nasal mucosa usually indicates
- a) sinusitus
- b) recurrent epistaxis
- c) allergy
- d) acute infection

14 Nasal polyps, unlike the turbinates, are
- a) soft and mobile
- b) hard and vascular
- c) tender to palpation
- d) easily transilluminated

Adult

15 The number of pairs of paranasal sinuses present in the adult is
- a) 2
- b) 3
- c) 4
- d) 6

Pediatric

16 Which of the following sinuses are present at birth?
- a) maxillary
- b) ethmoid
- c) sphenoid
- d) *a* and *b*
- e) *a* and *c*

TRUE—FALSE

Adult and Pediatric

_____**1** The four sets of sinuses on each side are interconnected by air passageways.

_____**2** All four sets of sinuses are normally lined by an extension of the nasal mucosa.

_____**3** The opening between the turbinates is referred to as the choana.

_____**4** 90% of all nosebleeds come from a rupture of Kiesselbach's plexus.

_____**5** The nasolacrimal duct opens into the superior meatus.

_____**6** The superior turbinate is the largest, but is the most difficult to visualize.

_____**7** The olfactory region of the nose is located high on the nasal septum and superior turbinate.

_____**8** Another name for the maxillary sinus is the antrum of Highmore.

_____**9** A broad, flat "saddle" nose may be a sign of congenital syphilis.

_____**10** The nasal mucosa is less red than the oral mucosa.

PHYSICAL EXAMINATION: MOUTH AND THROAT

Behavioral Objectives

The student will be able to:

1 answer in writing all *Review Questions*
2 define in writing the terms listed under *Definitions*
3 identify and label the following anatomical structures on Figure 6–4: anterior tonsillar pillar, posterior tonsillar pillar, palatine tonsil, uvula, palatine arch, posterior pharyngeal wall, hard palate, soft palate
4 demonstrate the proper technique for examining the mouth and throat (including palpation and inspection)
5 accurately record the findings of an oral examination
6 identify and label the teeth illustrated in Figure 6–5 (deciduous dentition) and in Figure 6–6 (permanent dentition)
7 identify and label the various parts of the tooth illustrated in Figure 6–7
8 identify and label the three portions of the pharynx illustrated in Figure 6–8
9 identify various forms of malocclusion, dental decay, and periodontal disease at various stages, on clinical examination
10 answer the questions from frames 6.0–7.30 and pages 11–15 in *AJN* (May 1975) programmed instruction
11 label salivary glands as shown in Figure 6–9.

Figure 6–4
Structures in the mouth and pharynx

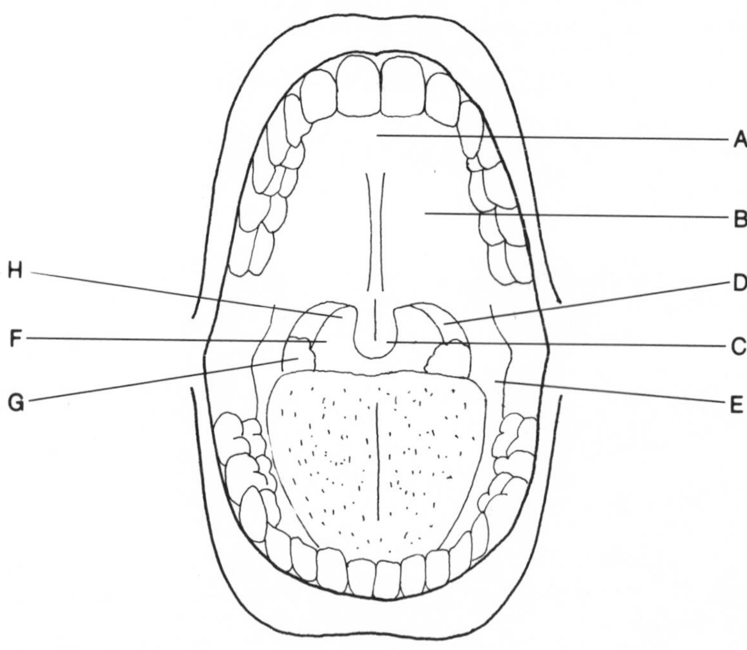

Label:

___**1. anterior tonsillar pillar**	___**5. palatine arch**
___**2. posterior tonsillar pillar**	___**6. posterior pharyngeal wall**
___**3. palatine tonsil**	___**7. hard palate**
___**4. uvula**	___**8. soft palate**

Learning Activities

Required

A *Read:* Alexander and Brown, Bates

B *View:* Blue Hill Series videotapes *Pediatric Examination—Ear, Nose, Mouth and Throat; Physical Assessment—Ear, Nose, Throat and Mouth*

C *Label:* Figures 6–4, 6–5, 6–6, 6–7, 6–8, and 6–9

D *Complete:* list of definitions

E *Complete:* programmed learning in *AJN* (May 1975): frames 6.0–7.30; pp. 11–15

F *Examine* the oral cavities of three children and three adults, using a mirror, and record findings on the check list provided.

Figure 6–5
Deciduous dentition

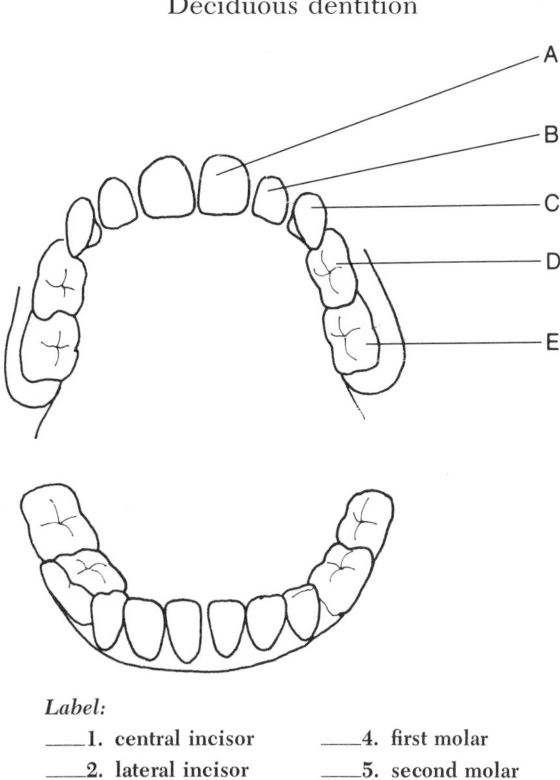

Label:

___1. central incisor
___2. lateral incisor
___3. cuspid
___4. first molar
___5. second molar

Figure 6–6
Permanent dentition

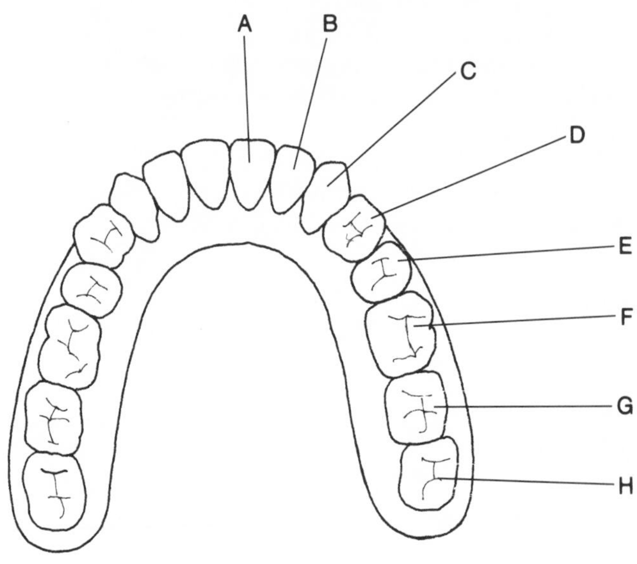

Label:

___1. lateral incisor
___2. central incisor
___3. cuspid
___4. second bicuspid
___5. first bicuspid
___6. first molar
___7. second molar
___8. third molar

Figure 6–7
Parts of the tooth

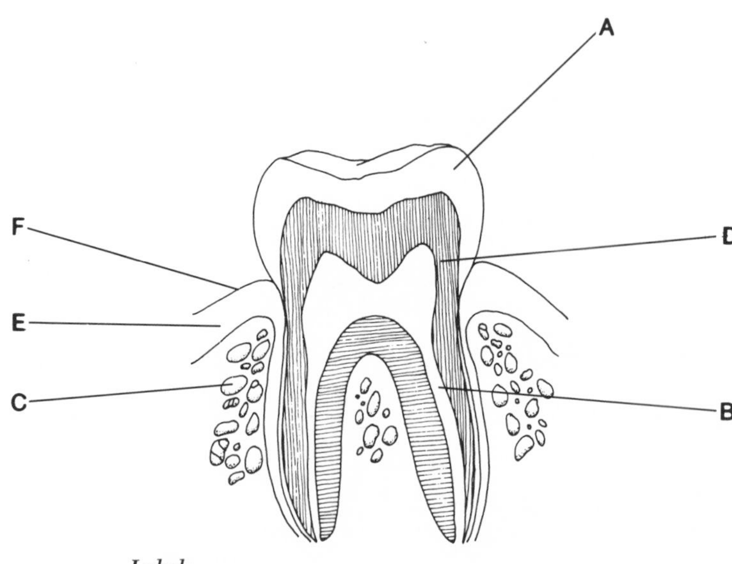

Label:

___1. enamel
___2. dentin
___3. pulp
___4. periodontal membrane
___5. gingiva
___6. bone

Figure 6–8
Divisions of the pharynx

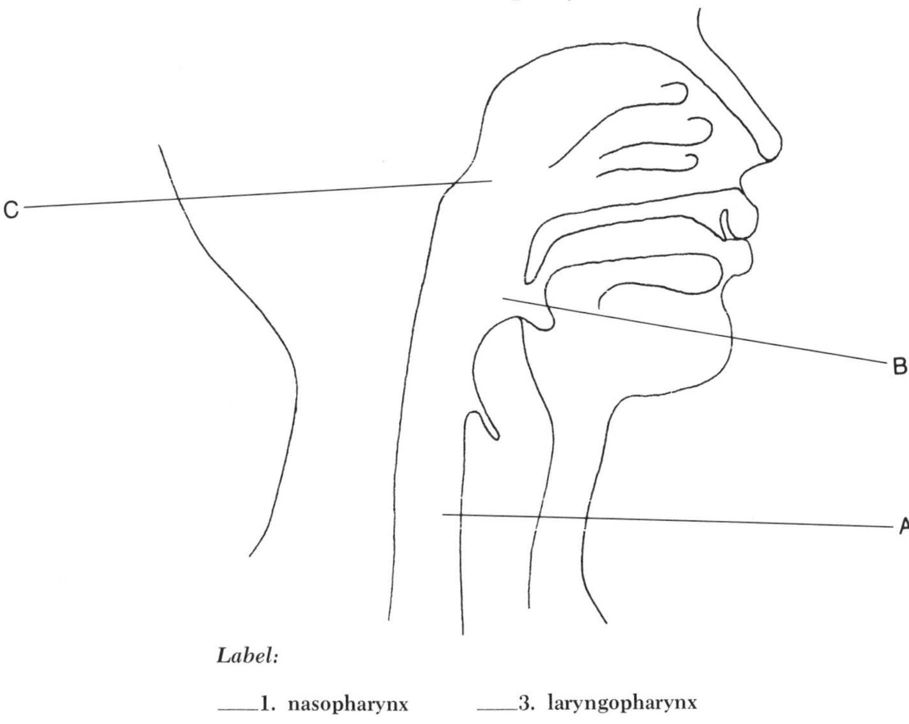

Label:

____1. nasopharynx

____2. oropharynx

____3. laryngopharynx

Figure 6–9

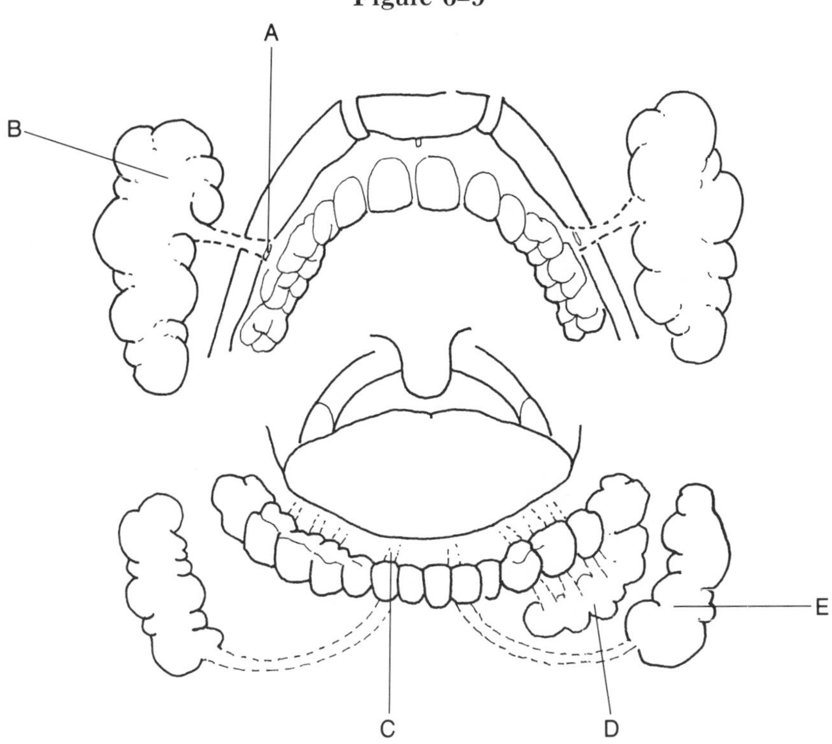

Label:

____1. parotid gland

____2. submandibular gland

____3. sublingual gland

____4. Wharton's duct opening

____5. Stensen's duct opening

Definitions

Match the definitions in *Column I* with the correct words in *Column II.*

Column I		Column II
_____1	bald tongue; smooth, glistening tongue with atrophic papillae; observed in pernicious anemia and in the late stages of chronic recurrent pellagra	**A** papillae
_____2	localized, progressively destructive disease of the teeth that starts at the external surface (enamel) with the apparent dissolution of the inorganic components by organic acids	**B** leukoplakia
_____3	difficulty in swallowing	**C** halitosis
_____4	toothless; without teeth	**D** atrophic glossitis
_____5	a saddle-shaped plate of cartilage covered with mucous membrane, at the root of the tongue, which folds back over the aperture of the larynx, covering it during the act of swallowing	**E** glossoptosis
_____6	small, white epithelial masses on the palate of the newborn; considered normal	**F** periodontitis
_____7	a fold of mucous membrane extending from the floor of the mouth to the midline of the undersurface of the tongue	**G** micrognathia
_____8	the occurrence on the dorsum of the tongue of peripherally spreading patches of temporary papillary atrophy; transitory, benign migrating plaques; coalescence of the lesions produces an irregular, maplike appearance	**H** Hutchinson's teeth
_____9	inflammation of the gums	**I** hard palate
_____10	inflammation of the tongue	**J** caries
_____11	displacement of the tongue forward	**K** gingivitis
_____12	bad breath; often caused by poor dental hygiene	**L** thrush
_____13	anterior part of the palate, consisting of the bony palate covered above by the mucous membrane of the floor of the nose and below by the mucoperiosteum of the roof of the mouth	**M** raspberry tongue
_____14	a virus infection marked by the eruption of one or more groups of vesicles on the lips or at the external nares	**N** herpes simplex
_____15	the teeth associated with congenital syphilis; the incisal edge is notched and narrower than the cervical area	**O** dysphagia
_____16	formation of white spots or patches on the mucous membrane of the tongue or cheek	**P** glossitis
_____17	one of numerous elongated conical projections on the dorsum of the tongue, especially at the sides and tip	**Q** strawberry tongue
		R edentulous
		S geographic tongue
		T epiglottis
		U frenulum
		V Epstein's pearls

____**18** a disease of the periodontium, evidenced by inflammation of the gingivae, resorption of the alveolar bone, degeneration of the periodontal membrane, migration of the epithelial attachment apically, and formation of periodontal pockets

____**19** a tongue with a whitish coat through which the enlarged papillae project as red points, characteristic of scarlet fever

____**20** infection of the oral tissues with *Candida albicans* (yeast organism)

____**21** smallness of the jaws, especially the underjaw

____**22** a beefy-red tongue due to the desquamation of papillae filiformes

CHECK LIST

Physical Examination: Mouth and Throat

	Yes	No	Describe
Lips			
color normal			
fissures			
Oral mucosa and gingiva			
color normal			
lesions			
gums swollen			
gums sensitive to pressure			
gums bleeding			
gums discolored (e.g., a "lead line" or blue)			
irritated areas			
chancres			
white patches			
mouth breathing			
other			
Tongue			
papillae normal			
coating			
frenulum intact			
projection without tremors			
movement bilaterally			
can touch lower lip			
size normal			
geographic tongue			
texture (furrowed, smooth)			
color (white, beefy-red, cyanotic)			
Palate			
hard			
soft—notched?			
uvula			
length normal			
bifid			
elevates bilaterally on phonation			

	Yes	No	Describe
Tonsils			
palatine			
size normal			
exudate			
adenoids			
visible			
exudate			
lingual			
visible			
exudate			
Salivation			
amount normal			
ducts normal			
Stenson's			
Wharton's			
glands normal			
parotid			
submandibular (submaxillary)			
sublingual			
Dentition			
occlusion normal			
caries			
color normal			
dentures			

Review Questions

Adult and Pediatric

1 The condition in which the lips are cracked and bleeding is referred to as ___________.

2 Salivary glands are (exocrine/endocrine) glands.

3 Grinding of the teeth is known as ___________.

4 White, cheesy patches on the tongue and buccal mucosa that bleed when removed are likely to be ___________.

5 A green or black discoloration of the teeth usually comes from ___________, which is a (temporary/permanent) condition.

6 A beefy-red, swollen tongue is associated with ___________.

7 Squamous cell carcinoma may appear as a (tender/nontender) lesion on the lips or tongue.

8 Tongue-tie is defined as a tongue that cannot be extended as far as the ___________.

9 Stensen's duct has an inflamed and edematous appearance in ___________. (name of disease)

10 A bony protuberance or exostosis in the midline of the palate is referred to as a ___________.

11 A patient whose breath has a sweet, acetone-like odor may be in a state of ___________.

Pediatric

12 A child is expected to get ___________ deciduous teeth.

13 Tetracycline can discolor a child's permanent teeth if administered anytime from ___________ to ___________ years of age.

14 A child usually begins shedding his deciduous teeth at approximately ___________.

Adult

15 An adult is expected to have ___________ permanent teeth.

Multiple Choice

(Mark the correct answer or answers)

Adult and Pediatric

1 The normal mucous membranes of the mouth structures should have all of the following characteristics except
- a) bright pink color
- b) moistness
- c) shininess
- d) irregular appearance

2 The tonsils that are usually visible when swollen are the
- a) lingual tonsils
- b) palatine tonsils
- c) pharyngeal tonsils
- d) adenoids

3 The adenoids are located in the
- a) oropharynx
- b) nasopharynx
- c) near the epiglottis
- d) laryngopharynx

4 Three important signs of tonsillitis are
- a) swollen tonsils
- b) a cold
- c) redness in the surrounding structures
- d) fever

5 The main reason why a patient with pharyngitis must be given prompt medical attention is that
- a) a broad-spectrum antibiotic must be prescribed
- b) his pain requires treatment
- c) pharyngitis is frequently the precursor of a more serious condition
- d) his condition is probably communicable

6 Infections involving the adenoids and complications from such infections are most common in
- a) infants
- b) young children
- c) young adults
- d) middle-aged people

7 In examining the salivary glands, you should be alert primarily to
- a) swelling
- b) signs of inflammation
- c) whether the gland is located in the normal place
- d) how well they secrete saliva

8 All of the following are possible causes of halitosis except
- a) foreign object in nose
- b) poor oral hygiene
- c) dehydration
- d) bruxism

9 Mottled and pitted teeth are seen in individuals who have been exposed to excess amounts of
- a) fluoride
- b) tetracycline
- c) x-ray
- d) oral iron

10 Possible causes of gingival hypertrophy are
- a) Dilantin
- b) gingivitis
- c) smoking
- d) all the above

11 Melanin pigmentation of the lips and buccal mucosa occurs in
- a) pernicious anemia
- b) Hodgkin's disease
- c) Addison's disease
- d) none of the above

12 Bifurcation of the uvula is associated with
- a) hearing loss
- b) absence of palatine tonsils
- c) submucous cleft
- d) delayed dental eruption

Pediatric

13 An increase in salivation usually occurs at approximately
- a) 2 months of age
- b) 3 months of age
- c) 4 months of age
- d) 5 months of age

14 The deciduous teeth usually begin erupting around
- a) the 8th month
- b) sometime after the first birthday
- c) the 3rd month
- d) the 6th month

15 Koplik's spots, which appear as grains of salt on the buccal mucosa, are diagnostic of
- a) rubella
- b) rubeola
- c) herpes simplex
- d) thrush

16 The most prevalent of childhood diseases is
- a) measles
- b) chickenpox
- c) dental caries
- d) herpes simplex

Self-Evaluation Key

FIGURE 6–1 (p. 64)

1. E
2. F
3. C
4. D
5. A
6. B
7. G

DEFINITIONS—NOSE (p. 65)

1. D
2. G
3. E
4. B
5. F
6. A
7. C

FIGURE 6–2 (p. 65)

1. D
2. C
3. A
4. B

FIGURE 6–3 (p. 66)

1. D
2. C
3. B
4. A

REVIEW QUESTIONS—NOSE (pp. 68, 69)

1. e
2. b
3. b
4. a
5. b
6. a
7. d
8. d
9. d
10. c
11. d
12. e
13. c
14. a
15. c
16. d

TRUE—FALSE (p. 69)

1. T
2. T
3. F
4. T
5. F
6. F
7. T
8. T
9. T
10. F

FIGURE 6–4 (p. 70)

1. E
2. D
3. G
4. C
5. H
6. F
7. A
8. B

FIGURE 6–5 (p. 71)

1. A
2. B
3. C
4. D
5. E

FIGURE 6–6 (p. 72)

1. B
2. A
3. C
4. E
5. D
6. F
7. G
8. H

FIGURE 6–7 (p. 72)

1. A
2. D
3. B
4. F
5. E
6. C

FIGURE 6–8 (p. 73)

1. C
2. B
3. A

FIGURE 6–9 (p. 73)

1. B
2. E
3. D
4. C
5. A

DEFINITIONS—MOUTH AND THROAT (pp. 74–75)

1. D
2. J
3. O
4. R
5. T
6. V
7. U
8. S
9. K
10. P
11. E
12. C
13. I
14. N
15. H
16. B
17. A
18. F
19. Q
20. L
21. G
22. M

REVIEW QUESTIONS—MOUTH AND THROAT (p. 78)

1. cheilitis
2. exocrine
3. bruxism
4. thrush
5. oral iron, temporary
6. vitamin deficiency
7. nontender
8. alveolar ridge
9. mumps
10. torus palatinus
11. diabetic acidosis
12. 20
13. 2–15
14. six
15. 32

MULTIPLE CHOICE (pp. 78, 79, 80)

1. d
2. b
3. b
4. a, c, d
5. c
6. b
7. a, b
8. d
9. b
10. d
11. c
12. c
13. b
14. d
15. b
16. c

7

chest and lungs

TO THE STUDENT

It should be noted that the physical examination of the adult female breast is not included in this section, but will be covered in Section 9. You may want to combine *Learning Activity C* of the *Inspection* segment with *Learning Activity E* of the *Percussion* segment, *Learning Activity C* of the *Palpation* segment, and *Learning Activity D* of the *Auscultation* segment.

Recommended materials:

1 Alexander, Mary, and Brown, Marie. *Pediatric Physical Diagnosis for Nurses.* New York: McGraw-Hill Book Co., 1974
2 Bates, Barbara. *A Guide to Physical Examination.* Philadelphia: J. B. Lippincott Co., 1974
3 Blue Hill Educational Systems, Inc. *Pediatric Physical Examination—The Respiratory System* (Videotape: 40 minutes)
4 Blue Hill Educational Systems, Inc. *Physical Assessment Examinations—Respiratory* (Videotape: 14 minutes)
5 J. B. Lippincott Co. *Visual Guide to Physical Examination—Thorax* (Film/videotape: 7:30 minutes)
6 Druger, George, M.D. *The Chest: Its Signs and Sounds.* Inglewood, Calif.: Humetrics Corp., 1973. Text/tape (pages 3, 4, and 45 are reproduced in this section on pages 83–85). To complete the segment on auscultation in this section, students must also listen to Tapes 5B, 6A, 6B, 7A, 7B, and 8A
7 access to three adults and three children willing to let you examine their chests

BASIC KNOWLEDGE

Behavioral Objectives

The student will be able to:

1 answer in writing all *Review Questions*

2 define in writing the terms listed under *Definitions*
3 identify the landmarks of the chest on the anterior, posterior, and lateral chest according to Bates
4 on the diagrams of breath sounds shown on pages 83–85:
  a) identify the line representing inspiration
  b) identify the line representing expiration
  c) state in writing whether inspiration or expiration is louder
  d) state in writing whether inspiration or expiration is longer
5 describe in writing the findings indicated in Figures 7–6 and 7–7
6 locate on the figure the findings described in Figure 7–8
7 identify by marking with a marking pen the following underlying structures of the chest (from front, back, and side—as in Bates
  a) trachea
  b) lobes of each lung.

Learning Activities

I Required
  A *Read:*
    1 Alexander and Brown
    2 Bates (paying particular attention to the diagrams)
  B *Study:* diagrams in Bates (anatomy and physiology of thorax and lungs)
  C *Complete:* Figures 7–6, 7–7, 7–8
II Optional
  See listing of additional references and materials specific to chest and lungs in *Bibliography.*

THE CHEST: ITS SIGNS AND SOUNDS*

The thickness of each line represents the amplitude or loudness of each part of the breath sound. In Figure 7–1 it can be seen that the thickness of the upstroke or inspiratory line is greater than the thickness of the downstroke or expiratory line. This indicates that the inspiratory phase is louder than the expiratory phase.

Figure 7–1
Diagrammatic representation of a normal breath sound

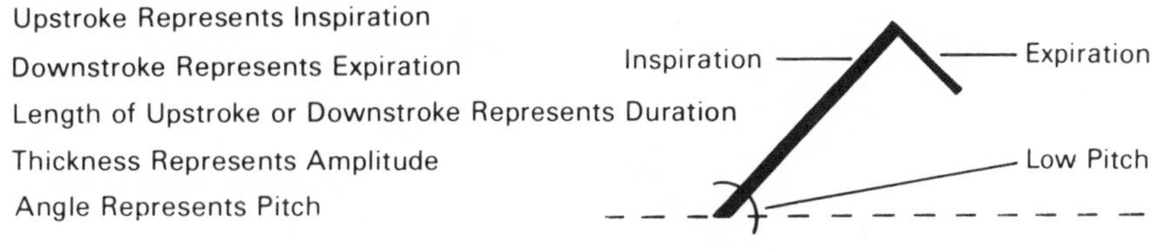

Upstroke Represents Inspiration
Downstroke Represents Expiration
Length of Upstroke or Downstroke Represents Duration
Thickness Represents Amplitude
Angle Represents Pitch
Inspiration
Expiration
Low Pitch

The angle the ascending or descending limbs make with the interrupted horizontal line is the schematic representation of the pitch or sound wave frequency of the breath sound. A greater angle indicates a higher pitch. Figure 7–2 is a diagrammatic representation of a breath sound in which the pitch is higher than the pitch of the breath sound that is represented by Figure 7–1. Notice that the angle the limbs make with the horizontal interrupted line in Figure 7–2 is greater than the similar angle in Figure 7–1 thus indicating the higher pitch of the breath sound in Figure 7–2.

*From *The Chest: Its Signs and Sounds*, by George Druger, M.D. (Inglewood, Calif.: Humetrics Corp., 1973), pp. 3, 4, 45. Copyright 1973. Reprinted by permission of Humetrics Corporation.

Figure 7–2
Diagrammatic representation of a high-pitched breath sound

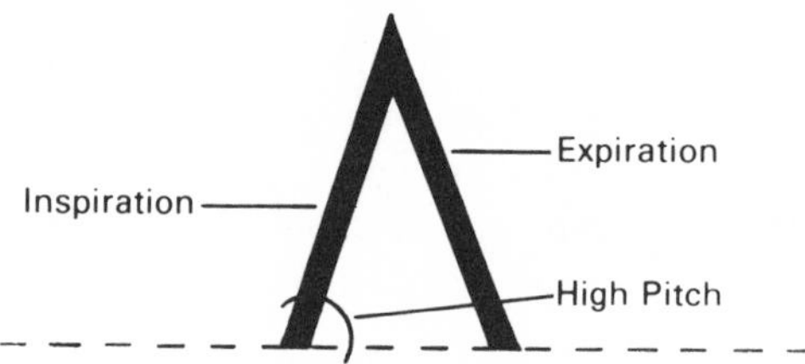

Figure 7–3 is the diagrammatic representation of a breath sound that has the same pitch and intensity as the breath sound diagrammed in Figure 7–1. However, the expiratory phase in Figure 7–3 is markedly prolonged as expressed by the length of the descending limb.

Figure 7–3
Breath sound with a prolonged expiratory phase

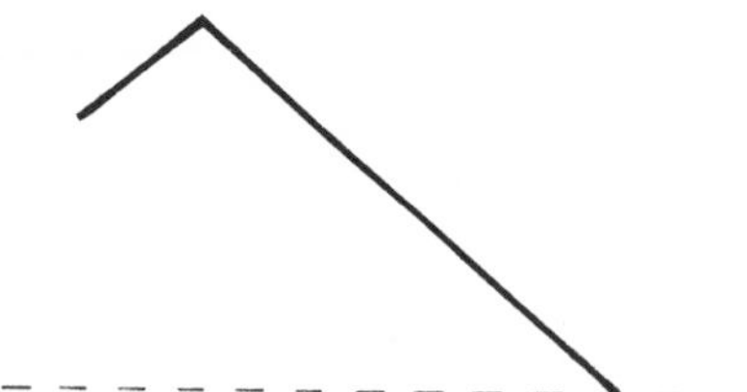

Figure 7–4 is the diagrammatic representation of a breath sound that has the same pitch and timing as the breath sound shown in Figure 7–1. However, the intensity or loudness of the breath sound diagrammed in Figure 7–4 is much greater, as reflected by the greater thickness of both the ascending and descending limbs.

In summary, the pitch, duration and intensity of every breath sound can be portrayed in diagrammatic fashion. This "shorthand" of describing breath sounds will be used throughout this text.

Figure 7–4
Breath sound with a loud inspiratory phase

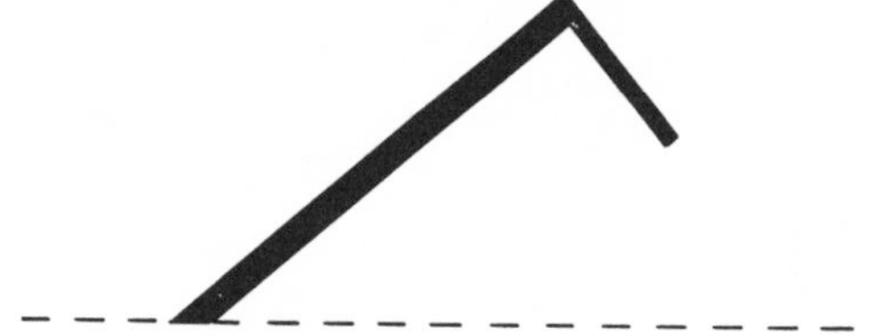

As you can see in Figure 7–5A, the inspiratory component is more intense, higher pitched, and longer in duration than the expiratory component. In the normal patient, the actual time consumed for expiration is slightly longer than the time consumed for inspiration, approximately in the ratio of 6:5. However, in the audible range of vesicular breath sounds, the ratio reverses and the inspiratory phase is heard approximately three times as long as the expiratory phase. During vesicular breathing, there is no pause between the inspiratory and expiratory phases of respiration.

Figure 7–5
Normal breath sounds

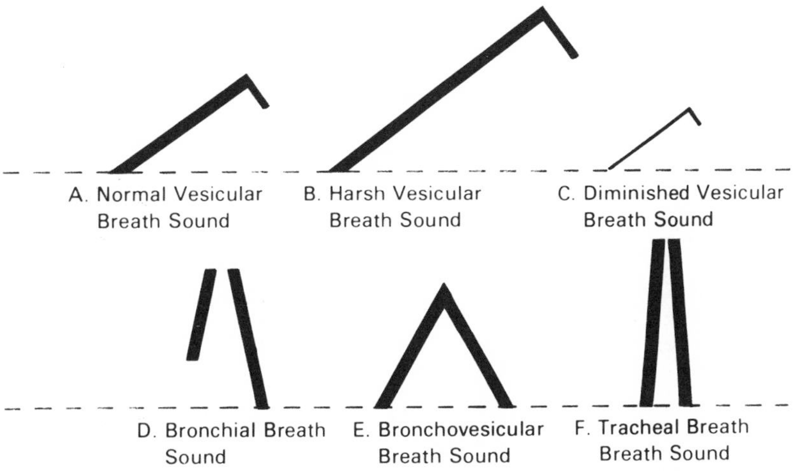

A. Normal Vesicular Breath Sound
B. Harsh Vesicular Breath Sound
C. Diminished Vesicular Breath Sound
D. Bronchial Breath Sound
E. Bronchovesicular Breath Sound
F. Tracheal Breath Breath Sound

Figure 7–6
Anterior view

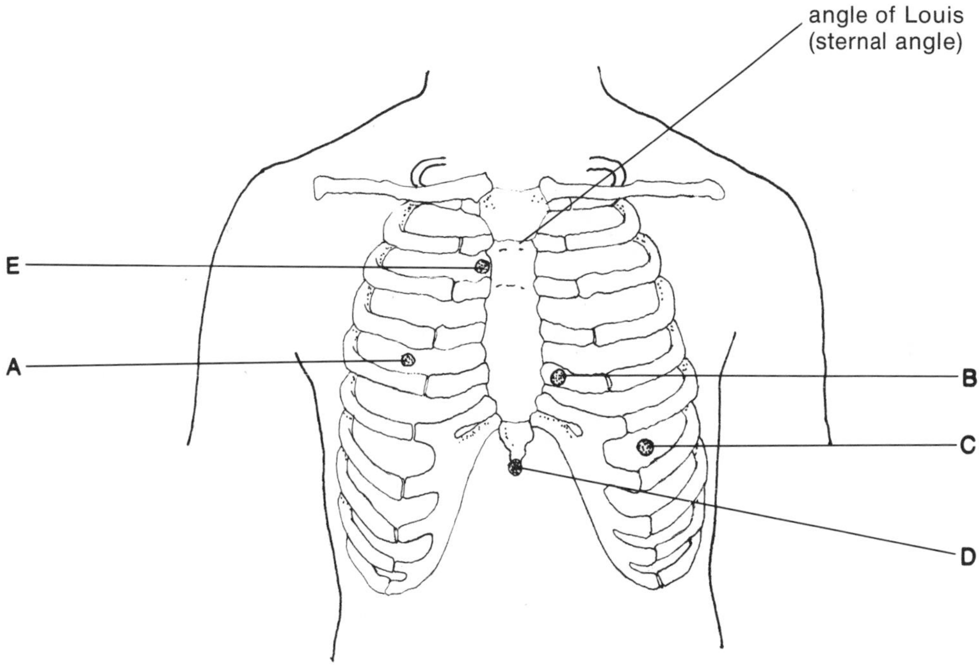

State below, in writing, the location of each finding shown on the figure (indicated by letters of the alphabet). This is the type of description you will be writing on a chart. Remember—be concise and precise. Do not use extra words, but be sure the person reading your description will know *exactly* where the finding is. *A* and *B* have been done for you, to serve as examples. The finding in all cases will be a 2 cm nodule. (See answers in answer key.)

A. a 2 cm nodule palpated at the 4th intercostal space in the right midclavicular line

B. a 2 cm nodule palpated at the 5th rib immediately adjacent to the left sternal border

C.

D.

E.

Figure 7–7
Left lateral view

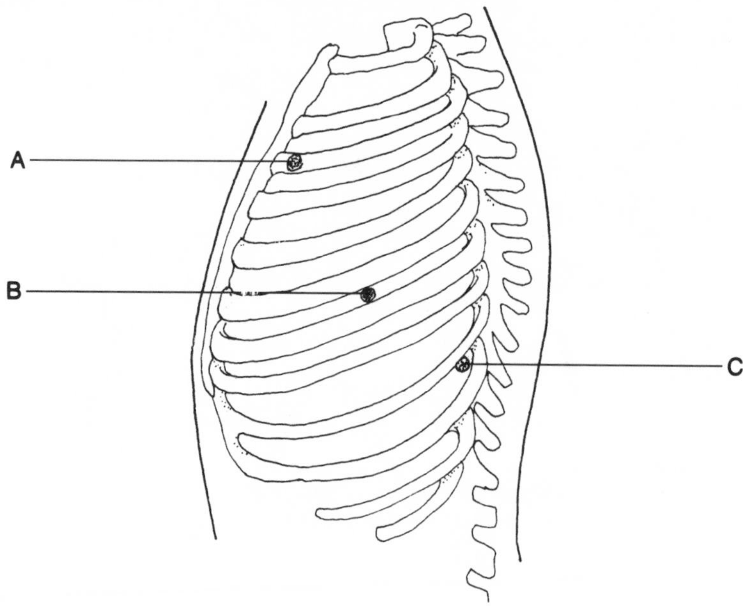

State in writing (as in Figure 7–1) where findings *A*, *B*, and *C* are located. Remember to use the landmarks you have learned. (See answers in answer key.)

A.

B.

C.

Figure 7–8
Posterior view

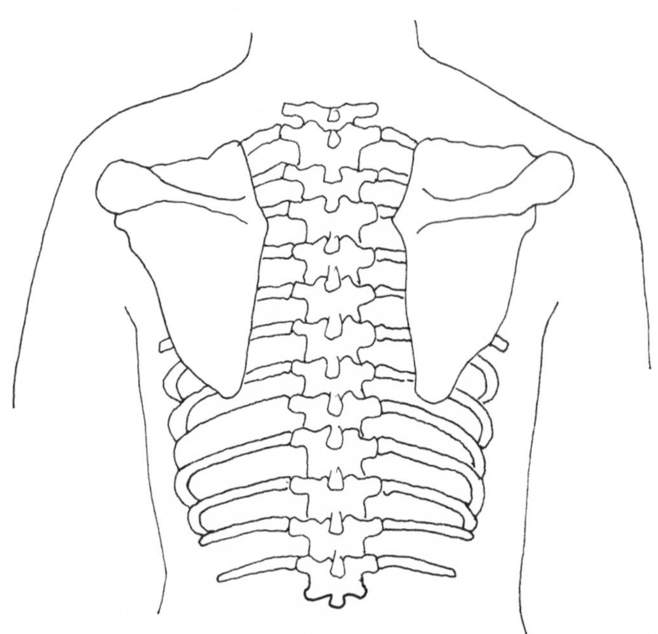

On the figure shown above draw in the findings at the locations described below. Each finding should be represented by a heavy circle linked by a line to the appropriate letter (as in Figures 7–1 and 7–2). Check your answers with the answer key.

A. a 2 cm. nodule palpated at the 8th rib in the left midscapular line

B. a 2 cm. nodule palpated at the 10th intercostal space in the midspinal line

C. a 2 cm. nodule palpated at the 9th intercostal space in the right midscapular line

Definitions

Match the definitions in *Column I* with the correct words in *Column II.*

_____1 this muscle's origins are the medial half of the clavicle, the anterior surface of the manubrium and body of the sternum, and cartilages of first to sixth ribs; its insertion is the crest of the greater tubercle of the humerus; its action is to adduct and rotate the arm

_____2 the air that is inspired and expired in normal quiet breathing

_____3 the greatest volume of air that can be expressed from the lungs after a maximum inspiration

_____4 a serous membrane enveloping the lungs and lining the walls of the thoracic cavity

_____5 the median dividing wall of the thoracic cavity, covered by the mediastinal pleura and containing all the thoracic viscera and structures except the lungs

_____6 the largest subdivision of the trachea serving to convey air to and from the lungs

_____7 one of the finer subdivisions of the bronchial tubes, less than 1 mm in diameter, having no cartilage in its wall

_____8 the air cells of the lungs; terminal dilations of the bronchioles where gas exchange is thought to occur

_____9 the upper part of the respiratory tract between the pharynx and the trachea; the vocal chords

_____10 pigmented ring surrounding the nipple

_____11 this muscle's origins are the anterior surface of the manubrium and sternal end of the clavicle; its insertions are the mastoid process and the occipital bone; its action is to turn the head obliquely to the opposite side and to pull the head downward and forward

A bronchi
B areola
C pectoralis major
D alveoli
E sternocleidomastoid muscle
F tidal air
G larynx
H pleura
I bronchioles
J vital capacity
K mediastinum

Review Questions

1 The apex of each lung is found about __________ cm above the inner third of the clavicle.

2 The right lung is divided into the right upper and right middle lobes by the __________ or __________ fissure, which runs from the right midaxillary line at the level of the __________ rib across anteriorly to the level of the __________ rib.

3 The trachea bifurcates into the two large bronchi at the level of the __________ anteriorly and of the __________ thoracic spine posteriorly.

INSPECTION

Behavioral Objectives

The student will be able to:

1 define in writing the terms listed under *Definitions*
2 answer in writing all *Review Questions*
3 label appropriately the sketches in Bates that illustrate normal thorax, kyphoscoliosis, barrel chest, pigeon breast, and funnel breast (as included under Deformities of the Thorax)
4 list in writing that four signs indicative of labored breathing are:
   a. suprasternal retractions
   b. flaring of the nostrils
   c. intercostal retractions
   d. tachypnea

Learning Activities

Required

A *Read:* Alexander and Brown, Bates
B *View:* Blue Hill Series videotapes *Pediatric Examination—The Respiratory System; Physical Assessment—Respiratory*
C *Examine and record findings:* inspection of the chests of three adults and three children of varying ages. (Use the check list provided.)

CHECK LIST

Chest and Lungs: Inspection

The following is a check list to be used by the student when doing the six chest and lung inspections required. Basically, there are three structures and one function in the area of the chest that can be assessed to some degree through inspection. Skin, muscles, and bones can be at least partially seen and must be included in the evaluation. Respiration is also an important part of this exam. The following list should be filled in for each inspection required in the learning activities (three adults and three children of varying ages).

Sex____________
Age____________

	Yes	No	Comments
Configuration Is this thorax: a barrel chest			
a funnel breast			
a pigeon breast			
Is the backbone: kyphotic			
scoliotic			
kyphoscoliotic			
lordotic			

Respirations

Rate____________
What is the normal for this age?____________
Rhythm: regular____________
irregular____________
Are they: abdominal____________
costal____________
What is normal for this age?
(abdominal or costal)____________
Is the depth:
normal____________
shallow____________
deep____________

Are there:	Yes	No
supraclavicular retractions		
substernal retractions		
intercostal retractions		

	Anterior	Posterior	Lateral
Describe skin			
markings (such as nevi, spider angioma, café-au-lait spots, etc.)			
color			
texture			
turgor			
hair distribution			
nipples			
Describe muscles			
symmetry			
hypertrophy			
atrophy			
symmetrical movement			
Bones visible			
deviations			
asymmetry			

Definitions

Match the definitions in *Column I* with the correct words in *Column II.*

Column I	Column II
____1 abnormal slowness of respiration	**A** tachypnea
____2 very rapid breathing	**B** bradypnea
____3 a chest permanently the shape of a barrel during full inspiration; seen in cases of emphysema	**C** Biot's respiration
____4 flattening of the chest on either side with forward projection of the sternum, like the keel of a boat	**D** Harrison's groove
____5 a hollow at the lower part of the chest caused by a backward displacement of the xiphoid cartilage	**E** barrel chest
____6 humpback; hunchback; an abnormal curvature of the spine, with convexity backward, due to caries and destruction of the bodies of the affected vertebrae	**F** pectus excavatum
____7 angular kyphosis	**G** funnel breast
____8 lateral curvature of the spine	**H** Kussmaul respiration
____9 kyphosis combined with scoliosis; severe congestive heart failure is not infrequently a complication	**I** pigeon chest
____10 a deformity of the ribs that results from the pull of the diaphragm on ribs weakened by rickets or other softening of the bone	**J** gibbus
____11 funnel breast	**K** kyphoscoliosis
____12 pigeon chest	**L** pectus carinatum
____13 the pattern of breathing characterized by a gradual increase in depth and sometimes in rate, followed by a decrease resulting in apnea; often associated with patients in terminal stages of illness	**M** kyphosis
____14 jerky and irregular respirations usually associated with increased intracranial pressure	**N** scoliosis
____15 deep, rapid respiration characteristic of the air hunger of diabetic coma	**O** Cheyne-Stokes respiration

Review Questions

1 What is the best position in which to place the patient whose chest is to be examined?

2 Normally, in a cross-sectional view of the chest the transverse diameter is __________ than the anterior to posterior diameter. (larger; smaller)

3 (Men; women) are more likely to have costal breathing.

4 Costal breathing in infants may suggest pathological problems in the (chest; abdomen).

5 List the six things that Bates states the examiner should look for in the chest while standing in a midline position behind the patient.
   1.
   2.
   3.
   4.
   5.
   6.

6 What should the ratio of the respiration to the pulse be?

7 What would the ratio of respirations to temperature normally be?

8 Bradypnea will (usually; seldom) necessitate a medical referral.

9 Name three observable signs of dyspnea.
   1.
   2.
   3.

10 The respiratory difficulties associated with kyphosis are usually quite severe. (true; false)

11 What is the scientific name for "hunchback"?

12 In what type of chest deformity are the ribs separated more than usual?

13 What is the most common cause of pigeon breast deformity?

14 Cheyne-Stokes respirations are (always; never) a sign of serious problems.

15 Biot's respirations would (always; never) necessitate a medical referral.

16 What is the most common cause of Kussmaul respirations?

17 If scoliosis has only one curve (i.e., one that forms a *C* rather than an *S*), it is more likely to be (functional; organic).

18 In metabolic acidosis, respiration is likely to be (increased; decreased) in depth.

19 In metabolic alkalosis, respiration is likely to be (increased; decreased) in depth.

Pediatric

20 A normal respiratory rate for an adolescent is 30 (true, false).

21 A normal respiratory rate for a newborn might be 30 (true, false).

22 An infant's respiration is primarily (abdominal, costal).

PALPATION

Behavioral Objectives

The student will be able to:

1 answer in writing all *Review Questions*
2 demonstrate the proper technique for eliciting vocal fremitus
3 demonstrate the proper method of palpating the trachea.

Learning Activities

Required

A *Read:* Alexander and Brown, Bates
B *View:* Blue Hill Series videotapes *Pediatric Examination—The Respiratory System; Physical Assessment—Respiratory*
C *Palpate and record findings:* examine three adults and three children, using the check list provided.

CHECK LIST

Chest and Lungs: Palpation

Describe all palpable findings in the skin, muscle, and bone of the thorax, being sure to locate them exactly according to interspace and/or rib. Do not forget to palpate the trachea for deviations. Include also your findings on tactile fremitus, respiratory excursion, costal angle, and costochondral junction.

Sex______________
Age______________

Review Questions

1 When testing for vocal fremitus, the examiner usually asks the patient to say __________.

2 In examining for tracheal deviations, the examiner should stand behind the patient and place his index fingers over the __________ to compare the space between the right clavicle and right border of the trachea with the space between the left clavicle and left border of the trachea.

3 Pneumonia would cause (increased; decreased) vocal fremitus.

4 Painful swellings of the first four costochondral junctions may indicate what syndrome?

PERCUSSION

Behavioral Objectives

The student will be able to:

1 answer in writing all *Review Questions*

2 label on Figure 7–9 the areas where percussion would be expected to be dull or flat; tympanic; resonant

3 demonstrate the proper method of mediate and intermediate (direct and indirect) percussion.

Learning Activities

Required

A *Read:* Alexander and Brown; Bates

B *View:* Blue Hill Series videotapes *Pediatric Examination—The Respiratory System; Physical Assessment—Respiratory*

C *Label:* the areas on Figure 7–9 indicating the appropriate percussion notes

D *Draw* the following organs on Figure 7–10 and indicate which ribs, interspaces, or other landmarks mark their borders: heart, liver, and spleen

E Practice percussing on three adults and three children of various ages and write up your findings on the check list provided. Draw the organs you percuss on the skin with washable marking pencil. See if they correspond to Figure 7–10.

Figure 7–9
Normal percussion notes

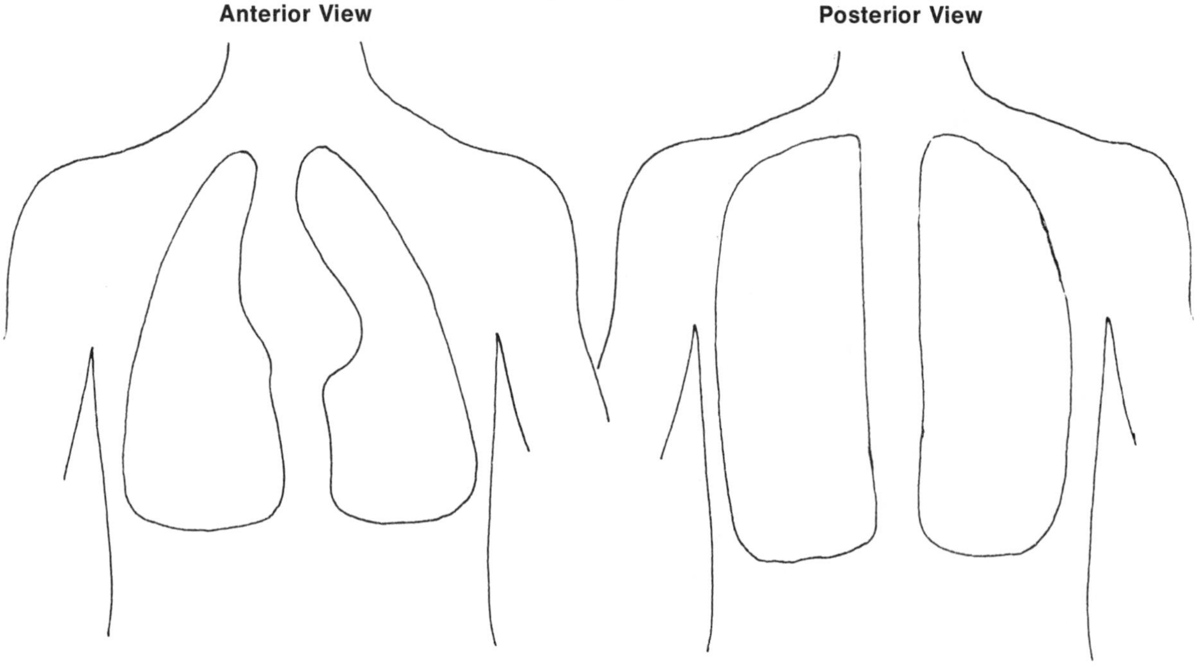

Color the appropriate areas in the diagram above to indicate where the four normal percussion notes are expected. Use the following color schedule:

1. **tympanic** ***(red)***

2. **dull** ***(green)***

3. **flat** ***(black)***

4. **resonant** ***(blue)***

Figure 7–10
Organs that can be percussed in the normal chest

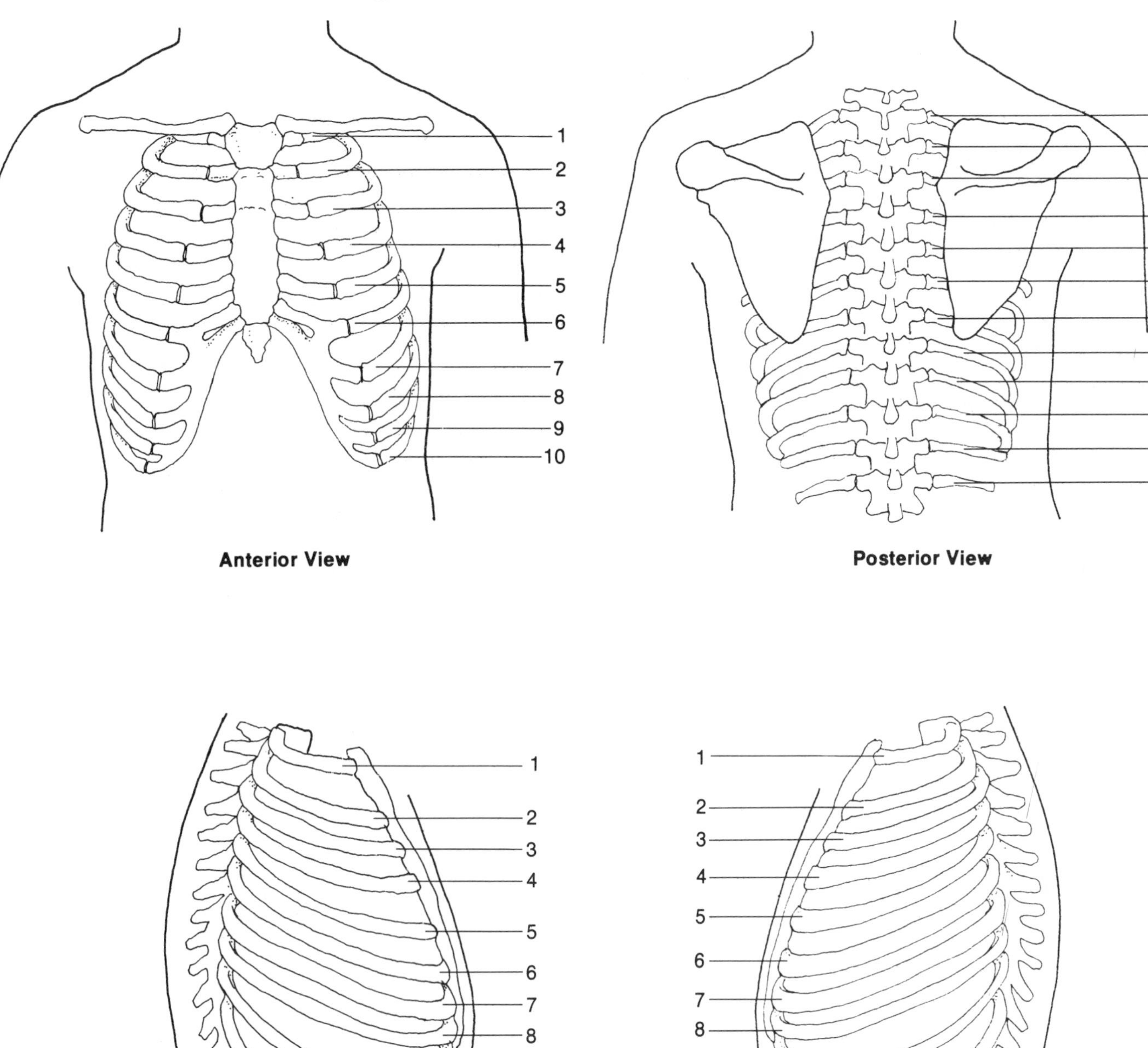

Draw in the following organs and list the interspace numbers or ribs that border them: ***heart, liver, spleen***

Review Questions

1 Describe the method of percussing for diaphragmatic excursion.
2 Symmetrical areas of a normal chest will never differ in the sound of their percussion notes (true or false).
3 The highest pitched of the percussion notes is __________.
4 __________ is the result of striking a hollow organ.
5 The only area in the chest where one would normally find tympany is over the __________.
6 Seven organs/structures expected to be dull or flat in the normal chest are: ____.
7 The normal diaphragmatic excursion is __________ cm.
8 A __________ or __________ percussion note will be heard over an area of the lung where air has been replaced by solid tissue or fluid.

AUSCULTATION

Behavioral Objectives

The student will be able to:

1 answer in writing all *Review Questions*
2 on a picture of the anterior and posterior thorax, color in the appropriate areas where he would expect to hear the three types of normal breath sounds
3 identify in writing tape recordings of the following: normal vesicular breath sounds, bronchial breath sounds, bronchovesicular breath sounds, tracheal breath sounds, normal voice sounds of the term "99," normal voice sounds of the letter "E," normal whispered sounds of "99," chest hair rubbing on the diaphragm of the stethoscope
4 identify in writing tape recordings of the following: harsh vesicular breath sounds, diminished vesicular breath sounds, asthmatic breath sounds, egophony, bronchophony, whispered pectoriloquy of "99," bubbling rales, gurgling rales, sibilant musical rales, sonorous musical rales, pleural friction rub.

Learning Activities

Required

A *Read:* Alexander and Brown; Bates
B *View:* Blue Hill Series videotapes *Pediatric Examination—The Respiratory System; Physical Assessment—Respiratory*
C *Color:* using appropriate colors, indicate on Figure 7–11 the areas where you would expect to hear the three normal breath sounds.
D *Listen to:* Tapes 5B, 6A, 6B, 7A, 7B, 8A (voice and adventitious sounds) in the Druger series.

Figure 7–11
Normal breath sounds

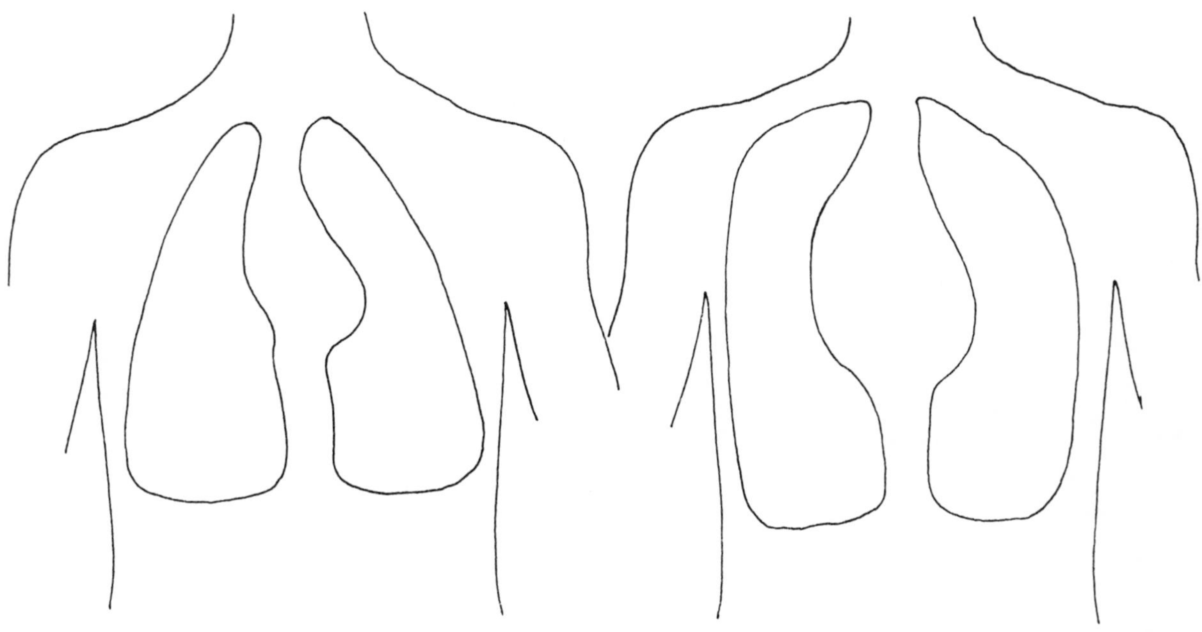

Color the appropriate areas for the 3 normal breath sounds

1. **bronchial** ***(blue)***
2. **bronchovesicular** ***(green)***
3. **vesicular** ***(red)***

CHECK LIST

Chest and Lungs: Auscultation

1 Describe exactly the area in which you heard the following sounds. (Be sure to include anterior, posterior, and both lateral positions.)

2 Describe any asymmetry of auscultation, explain it, and state whether it is normal.

Sound	Area	Is this sound normal in this area?		
		Yes	No	Describe; Explain
vesicular sounds				
bronchial sounds				
bronchovesicular sounds				
tracheal sounds				
rales				
normal voice sounds ("99")				
normal voice sounds ("E")				
sibilant rales				
sonorous rales				
crepitant rales				
subcrepitant rales				
bubbling rales				
asthmatic breath sounds				
egophony				
bronchophony				
whispered pectoriloquy				

Review Questions

1 Since most chest sounds are high in pitch, the __________ (diaphragm; bell) is used almost exclusively in the examination of the lungs.

2 Describe the proper positioning of a patient for examination of the chest and lungs.

3 Name two methods of avoiding the common error of mistaking a sound produced by chest hair rubbing against the diaphragm for breath sounds.

4 In what type of normal breath sound is the inspiratory component more intense, higher in pitch, and longer in duration (by a ratio of 3:1) than that of expiration?

5 In children, vesicular sounds are usually (more; less) harsh than in adults.

6 Diminished vesicular breath sounds are heard normally in the (upper; lower) portions of the lungs.

7 What normal breath sound is said to be "tubular"—like the sound of air passing through a hollow tube?

8 Bronchial sounds are usually (louder; softer) than vesicular sounds.

9 What normal sound might be mistaken for a pleural friction rub?

10 Breath sounds that are longer, louder, and higher pitched on inspiration and shorter, less loud, and lower pitched on expiration are what type of breath sounds?

11 Breath sounds characterized by a shorter inspiration and longer expiration are called what kind of breath sounds?

12 Breath sounds in which inspiration and expiration are equal in quality, intensity, pitch, and duration are called what type of breath sounds?

13 When alveoli are filled with fluid or tissue, bronchophony is (more; less) likely.

14 What is another abnormal breath sound found in the same condition as bronchophony?

15 In a normal chest you (would; would not) expect to hear a whispered word clearly through the stethoscope held over the chest.

16 An important principle of the physics of sound involved in auscultation of the lungs is that sound is transmitted (better; worse) through fluid and solid media than through air.

17 Asthmatic breath sounds have longer (expiratory; inspiratory) phases.

18 Musical rales are (continuous; discontinuous).

19 Two types of musical rales are: __________ and __________.

20 It is (true; false) that musical rales are always dry.

21 Wheezes are called (sibilant; sonorous) rales.

22 Sibilant musical rales are more common in the (expiratory; inspiratory) phase of respiration.

23 Sibilant rales are characteristic of what disease?

24 Sonorous musical rales are produced in the (alveoli; bronchi).

25 A musical rale most like a snore or groan is called __________.

26 Fine, moist rales are high pitched crackling sounds called __________ rales.

27 Crepitant rales are (discrete; continuous).

28 Crepitant rales are more likely to be heard during (inspiration; expiration).

29 Crepitant rales are most likely caused by the separation of the walls of the __________.

30 In patients who have been lying in bed for prolonged periods of time, rales similar to crepitant rales may be heard; however, these rales are less worrisome and disappear after several respiratory cycles. They are called __________.

31 Medium-moist rales are called __________.

32 Subcrepitant rales are thought to be caused by the separation of the adherent ________ walls.
33 Subcrepitant rales are more likely to be heard at the end of (expiration; inspiration).
34 Bubbling rales or rhonchi are (discrete; continuous).
35 Gurgling rales emanate from what part of the respiratory tract?
36 The nurse should expect to be able to understand clearly the syllables a patient whispers while she listens to the chest through a stethoscope. (true, false)
37 Egophony is (normal; abnormal).
38 A nurse would worry most about hearing (crepitant rales; bubbling rales).
39 Pleural friction rub (appears; disappears) when the breath is held.

Self-Evaluation Key

FIGURE 7–6 (p. 85)

C. a 2 cm nodule palpated at the left midclavicular line in the 6th interspace
D. a 2 cm nodule palpated at the lower edge of the xiphoid process in the midsternal line
E. a 2 cm nodule palpated at the right sternal border at the second intercostal space

FIGURE 7–7 (p. 86)

A. a 2 cm nodule palpated at the anterior axillary line at the 3rd rib
B. a 2 cm nodule palpated at the 6th interspace in the midaxillary line
C. a 2 cm nodule palpated at the 9th interspace on the posterior axillary line

FIGURE 7–8 (p. 86, see p. 104)

DEFINITIONS—BASIC KNOWLEDGE (p. 87)

1. C
2. F
3. J
4. H
5. K
6. A
7. I
8. D
9. G
10. B
11. E

REVIEW QUESTIONS—BASIC KNOWLEDGE (p. 87)

1. 2–4 cm
2. horizontal or minor fissure; 5th rib; 4th rib
3. sternal angle; 4th

DEFINITIONS—INSPECTION (p. 91)

1. B
2. A
3. E
4. I
5. G
6. M
7. J
8. N
9. K
10. D
11. F
12. L
13. O
14. C
15. H

REVIEW QUESTIONS—INSPECTION (p. 92)

1. sitting
2. larger
3. women
4. abdomen
5. deformation of the thorax; slope of the ribs; abnormal retraction of interspaces during inspiration; abnormal bulging of interspaces during expiration; asymmetry or impairment in respiratory movement; rate and rhythm of breathing.
6. 1:4
7. 4:1 (4 respirations for every degree over normal)
8. usually
9. flaring of nostrils; intercostal retractions; suprasternal retractions, cyanosis, subcostal retractions
10. false
11. kyphosis
12. barrel chest
13. rickets
14. always
15. always
16. diabetes mellitus, ketoacidosis
17. functional
18. increased
19. decreased
20. false
21. true
22. abdominal

REVIEW QUESTIONS—PALPATION (p. 95)

1. "99"
2. suprasternal notch
3. increased
4. Tietze syndrome

FIGURE 7–9 (p. 96, see p. 105)

FIGURE 7–10 (p. 97, see p. 106)

REVIEW QUESTIONS—PERCUSSION (p. 98)

1. See Bates, p. 88
2. false
3. tympany
4. tympany
5. stomach bubble
6. heart, spleen, diaphragm, scapulae, liver, kidney
7. 4–6 cm
8. dull or flat

FIGURE 7–11 (p. 99, see p. 107)

REVIEW QUESTIONS—AUSCULTATION (pp. 101–102)

1. diaphragm
2. sitting
3. press harder with diaphragm; wetting the hair
4. vesicular
5. more
6. lower
7. bronchial
8. louder
9. chest hair rubbing on diaphragm
10. vesicular
11. bronchial
12. bronchovesicular
13. more
14. bronchial, egophony
15. would not
16. better
17. expiratory
18. continuous
19. sibilant (wheeze); sonorous (snore)
20. false
21. sibilant
22. expiratory
23. asthma
24. bronchi
25. sonorous
26. crepitant
27. discrete
28. inspiration
29. alveoli
30. atelectatic rales
31. subcrepitant
32. bronchiolar
33. inspiration
34. discrete
35. trachea
36. false
37. abnormal
38. crepitant rales
39. disappears

Figure 7–8

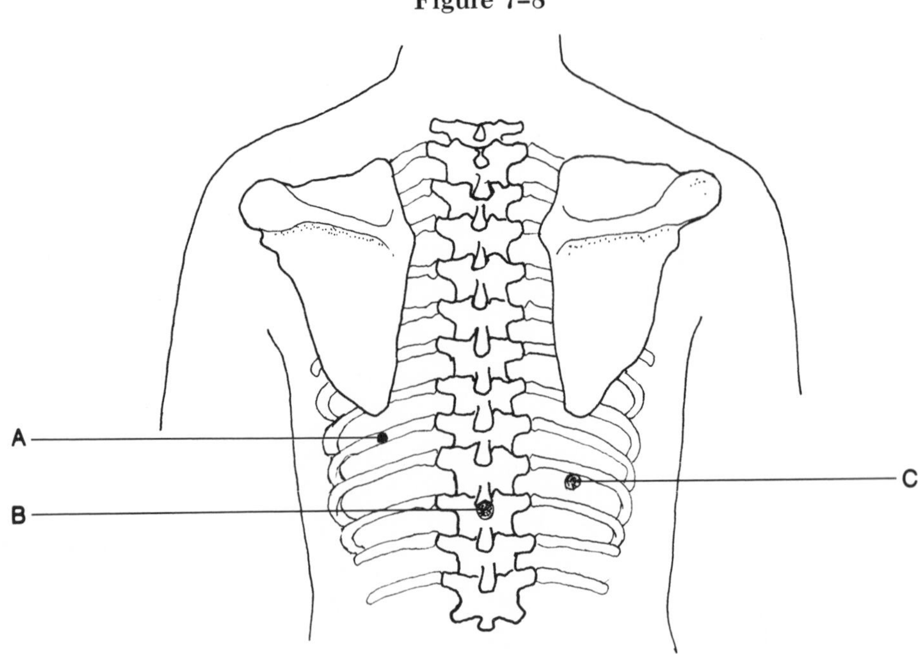

Figure 7–9

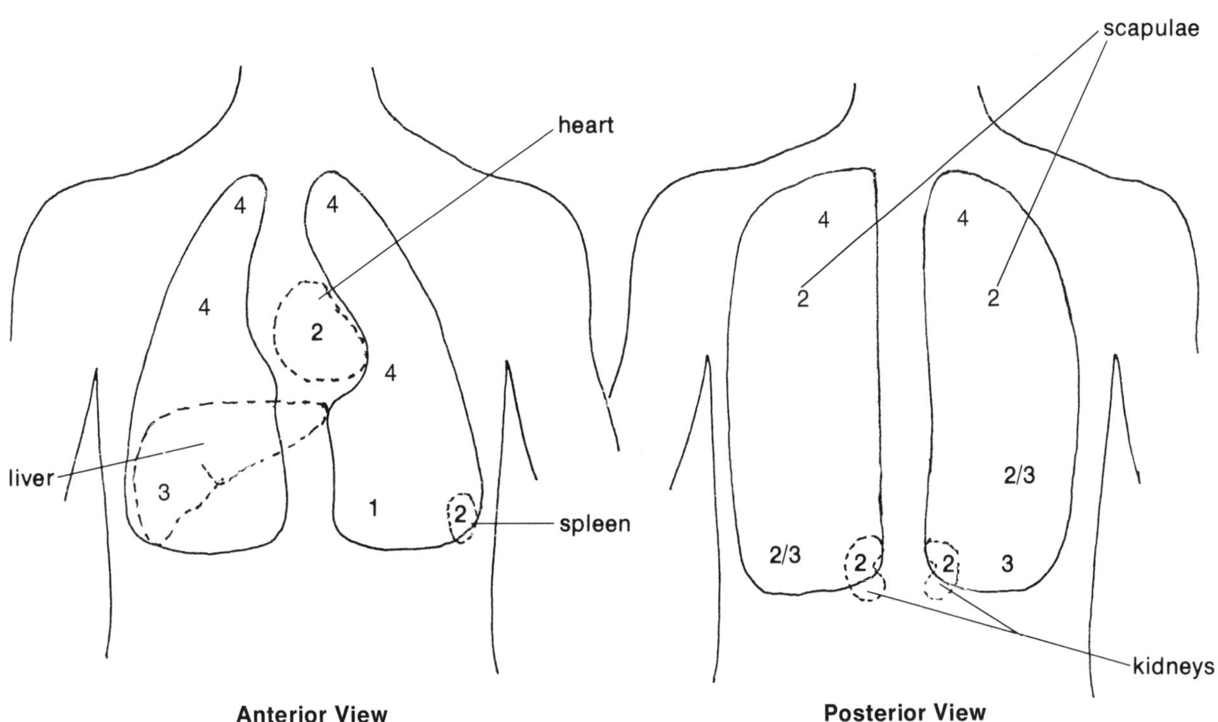

1. tympanic *(red)*
2. dull *(green)*
3. flat *(black)*
4. resonant *(blue)*

Figure 7–10

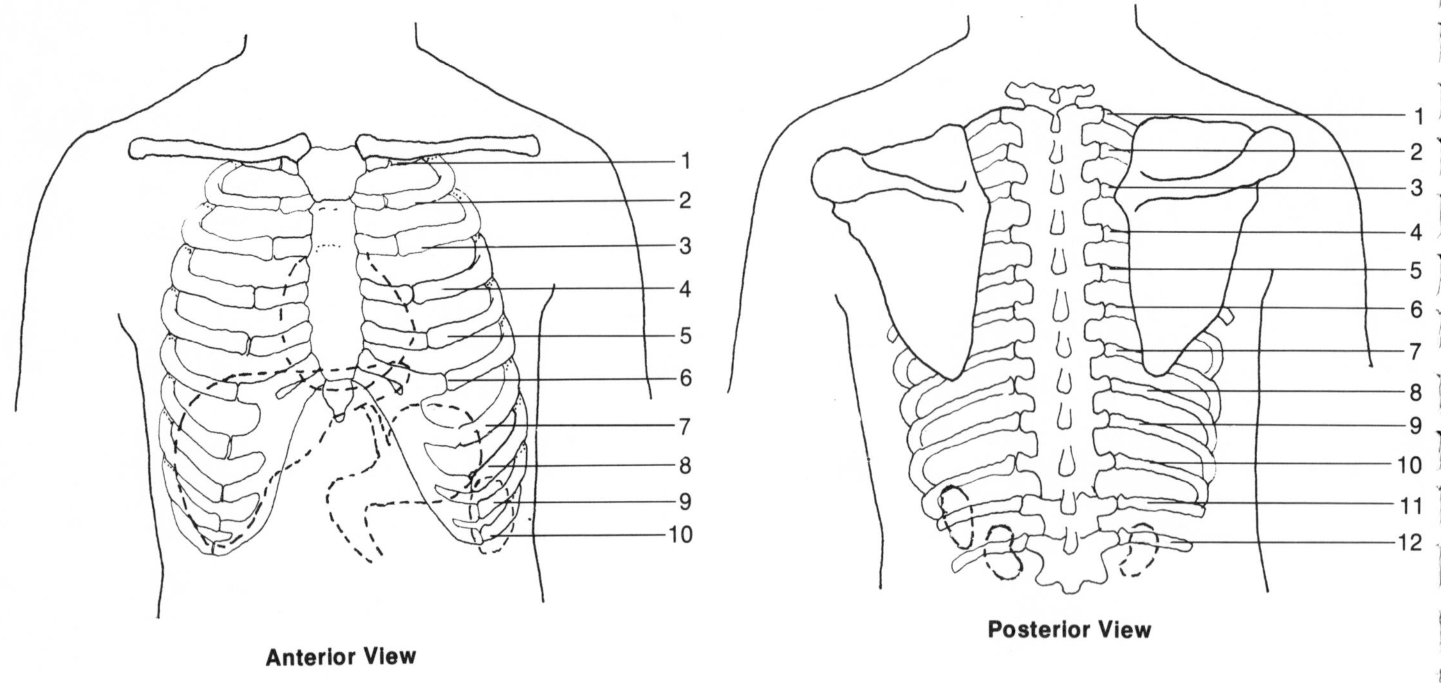

Anterior View

Posterior View

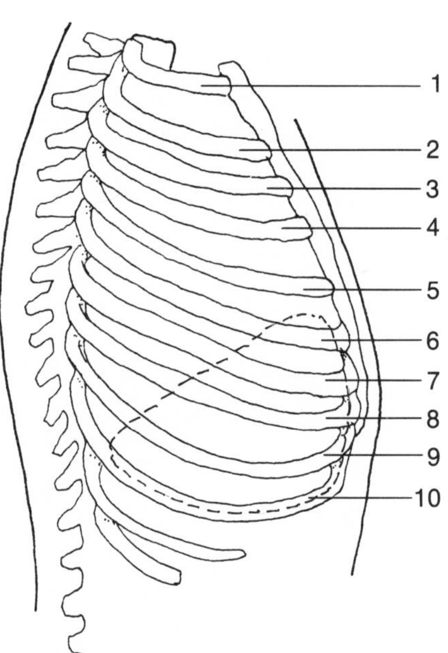

Right Lateral View

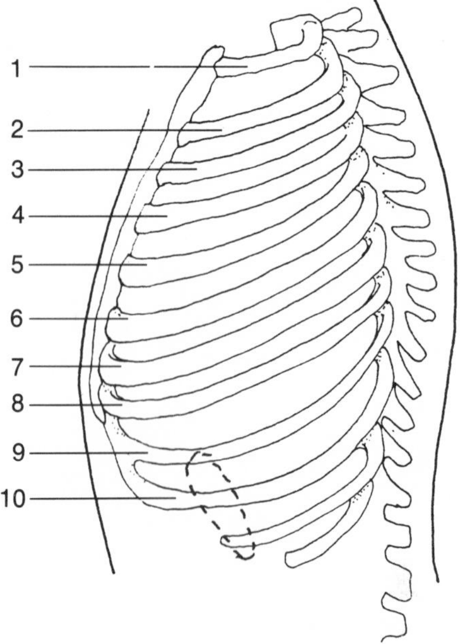

Left Lateral View

Figure 7–11

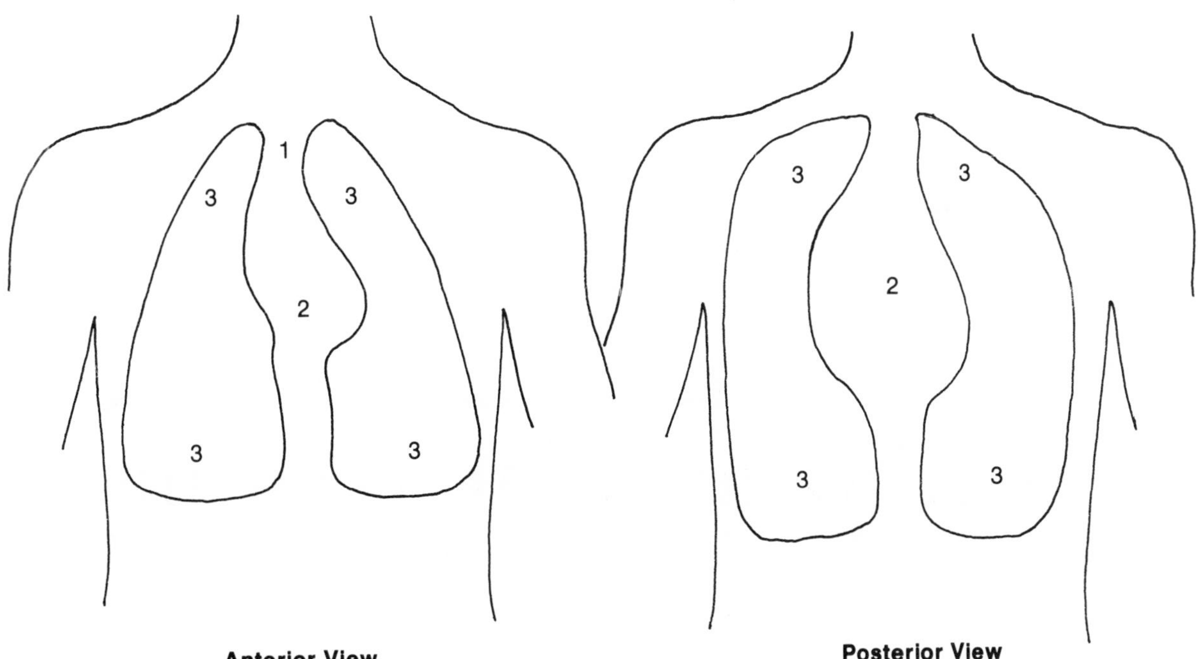

1. bronchial *(blue)*
2. bronchovesicular *(green)*
3. vesicular *(red)*

8

cardiovascular system

TO THE STUDENT

Learning activities from each segment *(Inspection, Palpation, Percussion, Auscultation,* and *Basic Knowledge)* involving examination of live subjects may be combined during the examination session.

Recommended materials:

1 Alexander, Mary, and Brown, Marie. *Pediatric Physical Diagnosis for Nurses.* New York: McGraw-Hill Book Co., 1974

2 Bates, Barbara. *A Guide to Physical Examination.* Philadelphia: J. B. Lippincott Co., 1974

3 American Heart Association. *Cardiac Failure in Infancy* (16 mm film; color, sound: 30 minutes). Shows physical signs found by careful examination; illustrates tachycardia, respiratory distress, sternal retraction, murmurs, cyanosis, and edema. Principles of immediate medical treatment for gradual or sudden onset of cardiac failure are presented.

4 Blue Hill Educational Systems, Inc. *Pediatric Physical Examination—The Cardiovascular System* (Videotape: 36 minutes)

5 Blue Hill Educational Systems, Inc. *Physical Assessment Examinations—Cardiovascular* (Videotape: 58 minutes)

6 J. B. Lippincott Co. *Visual Guide to Physical Examination—Heart* (Film/videotape: 6 minutes)

7 colored marking pencils (red and blue)

8 equipment: stethoscope
sphygmomanometer

9 access to at least three adults and three children willing to let you conduct a physical examination of their cardiovascular systems.

BASIC KNOWLEDGE

Behavioral Objectives

The student will be able to:

1 answer in writing all *Review Questions*
2 define in writing the terms listed under *Definitions*
3 trace the blood flow through the body via pulmonary and systemic circulation, using colored pencils as directed on Figure 8–1
4 label, in writing, the cardiac chambers, vessels, and valves, and trace the direction of blood flow through the heart as directed on Figure 8–2. Include the following:

left atrium
right atrium
left ventricle
right ventricle
aorta
inferior vena cava
superior vena cava
right pulmonary artery
left pulmonary artery
main pulmonary artery
pulmonary vein
pulmonary valve
tricuspid valve
mitral valve
aortic valve

Learning Activities

I Required
A *Read:*
Alexander and Brown (anatomy, blood flow, and conduction system of the heart); (glossary)
Bates (anatomy and physiology of the heart; study diagrams and illustrations carefully)
B *View:* Blue Hill Series videotapes *Pediatric Examination—The Cardiovascular System; Physical Assessment—Cardiovascular*
C Using colored pencils, trace the pulmonary and systemic circulation on Figure 8–1 as directed
D Follow directions on Figure 8–2 for labeling anatomical structures of and tracing blood flow through the heart
E Define in writing the terms listed under *Definitions*
F Answer in writing the *Review Questions*
II Optional
See listing of additional references and materials specific to cardiovascular system in *Bibliography.*

Figure 8–1
Pulmonary and systemic circulation

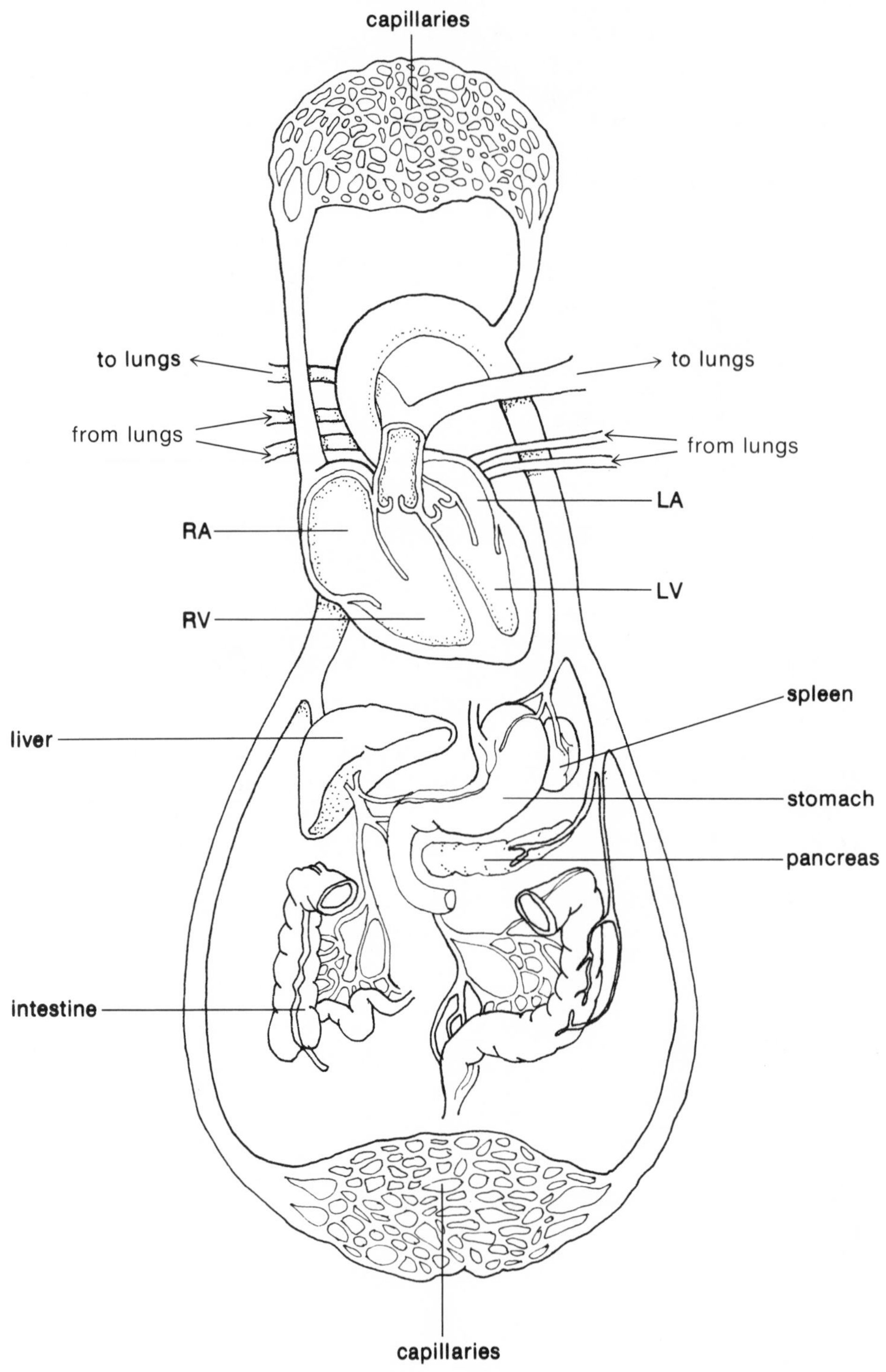

In the schematic diagram above, trace pulmonary circulation in *blue* marking pencil and systemic circulation in *red;* use *arrows* to indicate direction of flow.

Figure 8–2
Anatomy of the heart and adjacent vessels

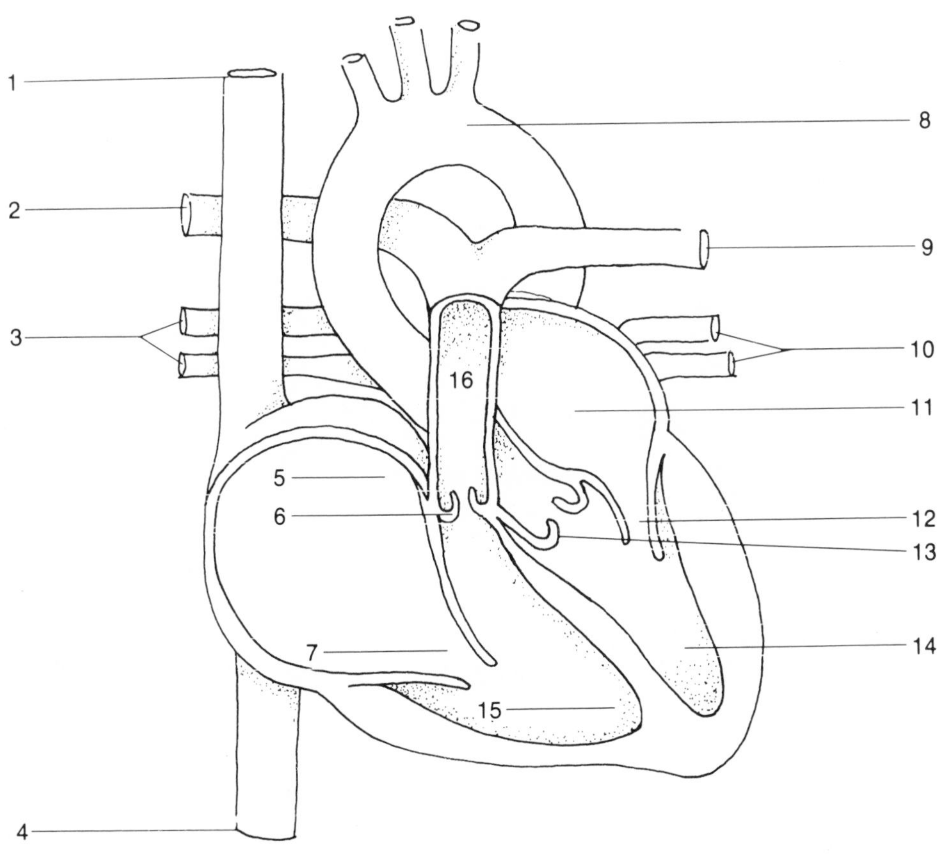

1. **Label the cardiac chambers, valves and vessels.**

____ left atrium	____ aortic valve	____ aorta
____ left ventricle	____ mitral valve	____ inferior vena cava
____ right atrium	____ pulmonary valve	____ left pulmonary artery
____ right ventricle	____ tricuspid valve	____ right pulmonary artery
		____ main pulmonary artery
		____ pulmonary veins
		____ superior vena cava

2. **Trace the course of oxygenated blood with a *red* marking pencil, using arrows to indicate direction of flow.**
3. **Trace the course of unoxygenated blood with a *blue* marking pencil, using arrows as above.**

Definitions

Match the definitions in *Column I* with the correct words in *Column II*.

____1 the upper chamber of each half of the heart, receiving the blood from the venae cavae on the right side and from the pulmonary veins on the left and transmitting it to the ventricle of the same side

____2 the left is a chamber of the heart that receives blood from the left atrium and drives it by contraction of its walls into the aorta; the right is a chamber on the right side of the heart that receives blood from the right atrium and drives it by contraction of its walls into the pulmonary artery

____3 the rhythmical contraction of the heart, especially the ventricles, by which the blood is driven through the aorta and pulmonary artery to traverse the systemic and pulmonary circulations, respectively

____4 the dilation of the heart cavities, during which they fill with blood

____5 irregularity of the heartbeat; loss of rhythm

____6 the part of the conduction system of the heart that leads from the A-V node to the ventricles; it passes within the membranous interventricular septum

____7 fibers found beneath the endocardium in the heart muscle; part of the combined structures that regulate heartbeat

____8 the visceral layer of the pericardium that immediately envelops the heart

____9 the innermost tissues of the heart, which include endothelium and subendothelial connective tissue

____10 the muscular substance of the heart, consisting of striated muscle tissue, differing somewhat from that of the voluntary muscles in that the fibers are shorter

____11 the membrane around the heart, the fibroserous membrane covering the heart and beginning of the great vessels; it is a closed sac having two layers—the visceral layer, or epicardium, immediately surrounding the heart, and the outer parietal layer, forming the sac composed of strong fibrous tissue lined with serous membrane

____12 the first heart sound; systole; synchronous with the carotid pulse

____13 the second heart sound; diastole

____14 one of the valves preventing regurgitation at the beginning of the aorta; a similar valve guards the entrance of the pulmonary artery

A systole
B pericardium
C palpitations
D atrium
E bradycardia
F endocardium
G ventricle
H tachycardia
I S_1
J diastole
K chordae tendinae
L tricuspid valve
M arrhythmia
N S_2
O Purkinje
P mitral valve
Q bundle of His
R semilunar valve
S epicardium
T myocardium

____15 left atrioventricular valve; bicuspid valve; valve closing the orifice between the left auricle and left ventricle of the heart

____16 right atrioventricular valve; valve closing the orifice between the right auricle and right ventricle of the heart

____17 the tendinous strands running from the papillary muscles to the margins of the atrioventricular (mitral and tricuspid) valves

____18 rapid beating of the heart, usually applied to rates over 100 per minute

____19 slowness of the heartbeat, usually applied to a rate under 60 beats per minute

____20 forcible pulsation of the heart, perceptible to the patient, usually with an increase in rate, with or without irregularity in rhythm

Review Questions

Part I

1 The electrical conduction system that controls the rhythm of heart contractility consists of the ________, ________, ________, and ________.

2 During ________ the aortic valve is open and the ventricle contracts, producing a ________ in pressure.

3 During ________ the mitral valve is open, the ventricle relaxes, and the pressure ________.

4 The first heart sound (S_1) is produced by closure of the ________ valve and tricuspid valve.

5 The second heart sound (S_2) is produced by closure of the ________ valve and the pulmonic valve.

Part II

Pediatric

1 The two most common cardiac problems in childhood are ________ and ________.

Adult and Pediatric

2 A third heart sound (S_3) may be produced by ________.

3 Occasionally one hears a fourth heart sound (S_4), which marks ________.

4 Three respiratory symptoms that may indicate cardiovascular difficulties are: ________, ________, and ________.

5 Symptoms of left-sided cardiac failure include ________, ________, ________, and ________.

6 Right-sided failure is characterized by ________, ________, and ________.

INSPECTION

Behavioral Objectives

The student will be able to:

1 answer in writing all *Review Questions*

2 define in writing the terms listed under *Definitions*

3 identify, by (1) labeling them on Figure 8–3 and (2) outlining them on a live subject, the seven specific areas on the anterior chest for cardiac examination:

1. sternoclavicular
2. aortic

3. pulmonary
4. anterior precordium
5. apical
6. epigastric
7. ectopic

4 identify signs and symptoms of cardiovascular disease that are evident from inspection of the patient, for instance:

cyanosis	edema—generalized
pallor	dependent edema
dyspnea	ascites
retractions	clubbing of fingers and/or toes
nasal flaring	abnormal PMI
precordial bulge	varicosities

Learning Activities

Required

A *Read:*

Alexander and Brown

Bates (focus on abnormalities detected by inspection)

B *View:*

1 Blue Hill Series videotapes *Pediatric Examination—The Cardiovascular System; Physical Assessment—Cardiovascular*

2 American Heart Association film *Cardiac Failure in Infancy.* Pay close attention to signs and symptoms such as cyanosis, pallor, dyspnea, precordial bulge.

C *Complete* Figure 8–3 by labeling the seven specific areas for cardiac examination

D *Define* in writing the terms listed under *Definitions*

E *Write* the answers to the *Review Questions*

F *Examine by inspection* the cardiovascular systems of three adults and three children. *Record findings,* using suggestions from the check list as a guide.

Figure 8–3
Inspection

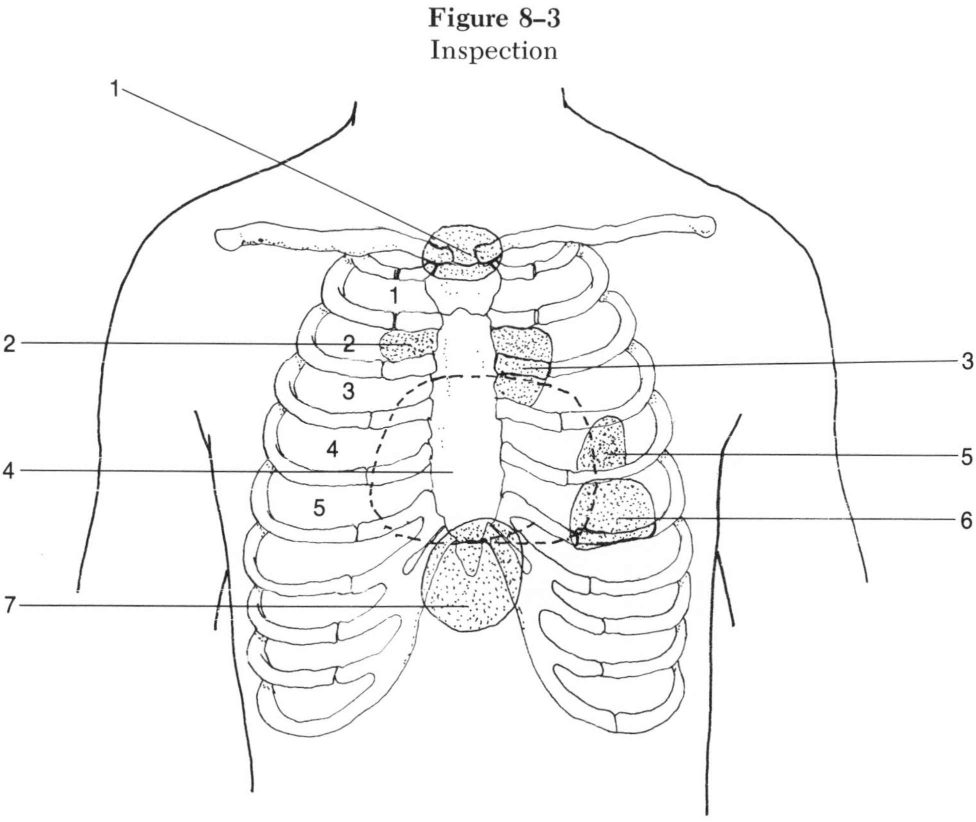

Label the seven specific areas for cardiac examination.

CHECK LIST
Cardiovascular System: Inspection

Describe all findings of visual observation related to the cardiovascular system.

Sex____________

Age____________

	Yes	No	Describe (*where appropriate*)
General behavior			
normal for age			
restless			
anxious			
irritable			
feeding poorly (infants)			
Respiratory status			
normal			
dyspnea			
orthopnea			
nasal flaring			
retractions: location			
severity			
respiratory rate			
Color			
normal for race			
pallor			
cyanosis: circumoral			
peripheral			
generalized			
at rest or when active			
Visible pulsations			
location			
intensity			
multiplicity			
timing			
Fluid stasis:			
edema (describe location and severity)			
ascites			
hyperemia			
venous stasis			
capillary refill			
Other abnormalities			
phlebitis			
precordial bulge			
PMI			
clubbing of fingers or toes			
varicosities			
scoliosis—left end bulge			

Definitions

Part I

Match the definitions in *Column I* with the correct words in *Column II.*

Column I	Column II
____1 difficulty or distress in breathing; frequently rapid breathing, usually associated with serious disease of the heart, lung, or nervous system	**A** generalized edema
____2 a dark bluish or purplish coloration of the skin and mucous membrane due to deficient oxygenation of the blood in the lungs or to an abnormally great reduction of the blood in its passage through the capillaries; it appears when the reduction of hemoglobin in the blood vessels is 5 mg or more per 100 ml	**B** point of maximal impulse
____3 a perceptible accumulation of excessive, clear, watery fluid in the tissues	**C** dyspnea
____4 edema of a body part that is hanging down or below the level of the heart	**D** peripheral cyanosis
____5 edema confined to a specific area, such as hand or foot	**E** localized edema
____6 edema that exists in the tissues of the entire body or of a large portion of the body	**F** cyanosis
____7 location on the chest of the strongest heartbeat; usually coincides with the apex of the heart	**G** edema
____8 the body trunk is a bluish or purplish color due to poor oxygenation; this indicates extreme conditions of poor oxygenation	**H** central cyanosis
____9 cyanosis of the more distal portions of the body, such as fingers and toes	**I** dependent edema
____10 paleness	**J** pallor

Part II

_____ 1 discomfort on breathing in any but the erect sitting or standing position
_____ 2 a protrusion in the epigastrium and anterior surface of the lower part of the thorax
_____ 3 broadening and thickening of the ends of fingers, seen in chronic pulmonary disease
_____ 4 depression, upon inspiration, of the skin particularly in the intercostal and substernal areas; seen in association with respiratory distress—especially in premature infants
_____ 5 dilated or knotted veins; enlarged and tortuous veins
_____ 6 the presence of an increased amount of blood in a part; congestion
_____ 7 an accumulation of serous, high-protein fluid in the peritoneal cavity
_____ 8 standstill or stagnation of blood in the veins
_____ 9 inflammation of a vein
_____ 10 inflammation of a vein with secondary thrombus formation
_____ 11 minute hemorrhagic spots, of pinpoint to pinhead size, in the skin
_____ 12 funnel breast; a hollow at the lower part of the chest caused by backward displacement of the xiphoid cartilage

A hyperemia
B precordial bulge
C pectus excavatum
D orthopnea
E varicosities
F petechiae
G clubbing
H ascites
I thrombophlebitis
J retraction
K phlebitis
L venous stasis

Review Questions

Pediatric

1 A slight retraction in the area of the anterior precordium may be normal. (true; false)

Adult and Pediatric

2 Cardiac impulse (PMI) is usually located at the __________.
3 A slight, brief, visible pulsation in the pulmonic area may be normal. (true; false)
4 Pulsations seen in the ectopic area may be normal. (true; false)
5 Examination by inspection should be done using __________ lighting.
6 Pulsations are most easily detected at the end of __________. (expiration; inspiration)
7 Bulging of the precordium is usually evidence of __________.
8 An excessive accumulation of serous fluid in the peritoneal cavity is called __________.
9 A left-sided bulge may not be due to heart disease; instead it may be a result of __________. (kyphosis; scoliosis)
10 Multiple pulsations in different intercostal spaces are usually the sign of __________.

Adult

11 A small bulge above the apex, animated by strong, expansive pulsations, is usually a sign of __________.

PALPATION

Behavioral Objectives

The student will be able to:

1 answer in writing all *Review Questions*
2 define in writing the terms listed under *Definitions*
3 demonstrate proper technique for palpating pulses and evaluating them with respect to rate, rhythm, character, and normalcy
4 demonstrate proper technique for palpating the anterior chest.

Learning Activities

Required

A *Read:*

1 Alexander and Brown (pulses)
(thrills and pulsations)

2 Bates (palpation)
(apical pulse)
(anatomy and physiology of blood pressure and pulse)
(arterial pulse)
(jugular venous pressure, abnormalities of the arterial pulse)

B Define in writing the terms listed under *Definitions*
C Write the answers to the *Review Questions*
D Palpate the precordium and pulses of three adults and three children and record findings, using the check list provided as a guide.

CHECK LIST
Cardiovascular System: Palpation

Sex______________
Age______________

	Palpable		**Symmetrical**		**Describe:** rate, rhythm, amplitude, contour
	Yes	**No**	**Yes**	**No**	
arterial pulses (bilateral) carotid					
radial					
brachial					
femoral					
popliteal					
dorsalis pedis					
posterior tibial					

	Identical		**Describe:** rate, rhythm, amplitude, contour
	Yes	**No**	
simultaneous radial and femoral pulse			

	Describe: utilizing skills of inspection and palpation
venous pressure	

	Locate: using anatomical landmarks		
cardiac impulse			

	Yes	**No**	**Describe:** in terms of location, transmission, and timing in cardiac cycle
thrills or abnormal pulsations			

hepatomegaly	**Describe**
pitting edema	**Describe**
ascites	**Describe**

Definitions

Part I

Match the definitions in *Column I* with the correct words in *Column II.*

____1 the angle formed on the anterior surface of the sternum at the junction of its body and the manubrium (central portion of the sternum, which articulates with the clavicles and the first two ribs)

____2 the difference between apical pulse rate and peripheral pulse rate

____3 if the blood volume is small and the artery can be easily obliterated, the pulse is feeble and/or weak

A pulse deficit

B thready

C sternal angle

Part II

____1 the vibration accompanying a cardiac or vascular murmur; can be felt by palpation; fremitus

____2 enlargement of the liver and spleen

____3 a perceptible accumulation of excessive, clear, watery fluid in the tissues which retain for a time the indentation produced by pressure

____4 a pulse regular in time, but with alternate beats stronger and weaker; often detectable only with a sphygmomanometer and usually indicating serious myocardial disease

A pitting edema

B thrill

C pulsus alternans

D hepatosplenomegaly

Review Questions

1 Cardiac impulse is usually palpated in the __________ left interspace, on or within the __________ line.
2 Palpable pulsations in the epigastric region may be normal in thin patients. (true; false)
3 Once a pulsation is identified, it can be time-linked to the cardiac cycle by __________.
4 Palpable pulsations in the ectopic area are __________. (normal; abnormal)
5 Venous pressure is __________ than arterial. (greater; less)
6 Three important determinations of venous pressure are:
   1.
   2.
   3.
7 The zero point from which venous pressure is measured during physical examination is the __________.
8 Explain how venous pressure is estimated, using inspection and palpation.

9 When palpating arterial pulses (especially radial or carotid) take note of:
   1.
   2.
   3.
10 When examining all cardiac patients it is important to include bilateral palpation of the following pulses:
   1.
   2.
   3.
   4.
   5.
   6.
   7.
11 Name two things that might cause an increase in pulse rate.

12 Are palpable pulsations in the epigastric region ever abnormal?
13 Thrills or vibrations in the aortic area should be referred for further evaluation. (true; false)
14 Systolic thrills in the apical area should be referred. (true; false)
15 Thrills usually occur as a result of __________ or __________.
16 Thrills should be described with respect to __________, __________, and __________.
17 Palpation of a pulsating liver indicates __________. (normalcy; abnormality)
18 Once a pulsation is identified, it can be time-linked to the cardiac cycle by __________.
19 In order to rule out coarctation of the aorta, the examiner should take the __________ __________ and __________ pulses simultaneously.

PERCUSSION

Behavioral Objectives

The student will be able to:

1 answer in writing all *Review Questions*

2 demonstrate skill in outlining the borders of the heart by percussing the anterior chest for cardiac dullness.

Learning Activities

Required

A *Read:*

1 Alexander and Brown

2 Bates (percussion)

B On Figure 8–4 of the anterior chest outline the borders of cardiac dullness as you would expect to percuss them in a normal adult

C Percuss the anterior chest of three adults and three children. Record your findings with respect to heart size and placement as outlined on the check list

D Write the answers to the *Review Questions.*

Figure 8–4
Percussion

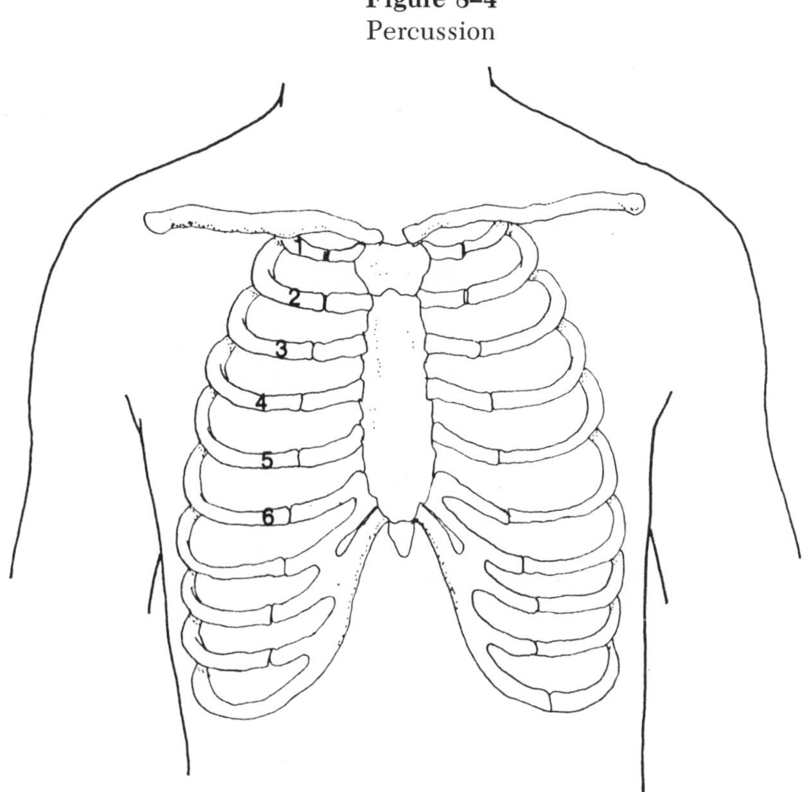

On the diagram above, outline the borders of cardiac dullness as you would expect to percuss them in a normal adult.

CHECK LIST
Cardiovascular System: Percussion

Sex______________
Age______________

Describe the area of percussed cardiac dullness, using anatomical landmarks. (A drawing such as Figure 8–4 might be helpful.)	
Are your findings normal?	
If not, how do you interpret them?	

Review Questions

1 In the cardiac exam, percussion of the anterior chest may reveal important information regarding heart __________ and __________.

2 What is the most important abnormal finding that percussion for cardiac dullness might detect?

3 Percussion usually reveals an area of cardiac dullness described by these landmarks:

AUSCULTATION

Behavioral Objectives

The student will be able to:

1 answer in writing all *Review Questions*

2 define in writing the terms listed under *Definitions*

3 identify verbally and/or in writing normal blood pressure measurements for infancy through adulthood

4 use cardiac auscultation to identify:
- a) the first and second heart sound
- b) the heart rate and rhythm
- c) splitting sounds of S_1 and S_2
  extra sounds in systole
  extra sounds in diastole

5 outline the seven areas to be examined when listening to the heart—on a diagram or on a live subject

6 list the five positions a patient should assume during a complete cardiac examination

7 state in writing whether he is listening to heart sounds at the apex or at the base (when blindfolded and listening to a live person)

8 identify the following heart sounds in writing and also diagram them, as they are heard on the recordings:
S_1
S_2
S_3
S_4

Learning Activities

Required

A *Read:*

1 Alexander and Brown (the stethoscope and auscultation)
(blood pressure readings)

2 Bates (auscultation)
(pay particular attention to content on murmurs)
(blood pressure)

B *Write* the answers to the *Review Questions*

C *Define* in writing the terms listed under *Definitions*

D *Label* Figure 8–5, which shows the relation of heart sounds to the chest wall

E On a live subject, *outline* the seven areas to be examined when listening to the heart. (If necessary, review *Inspection,* Figure 8–3)

F *Examine,* by auscultation, the cardiovascular systems of three children and three adults; record findings, using the check list as a guide.

Figure 8–5
Auscultation

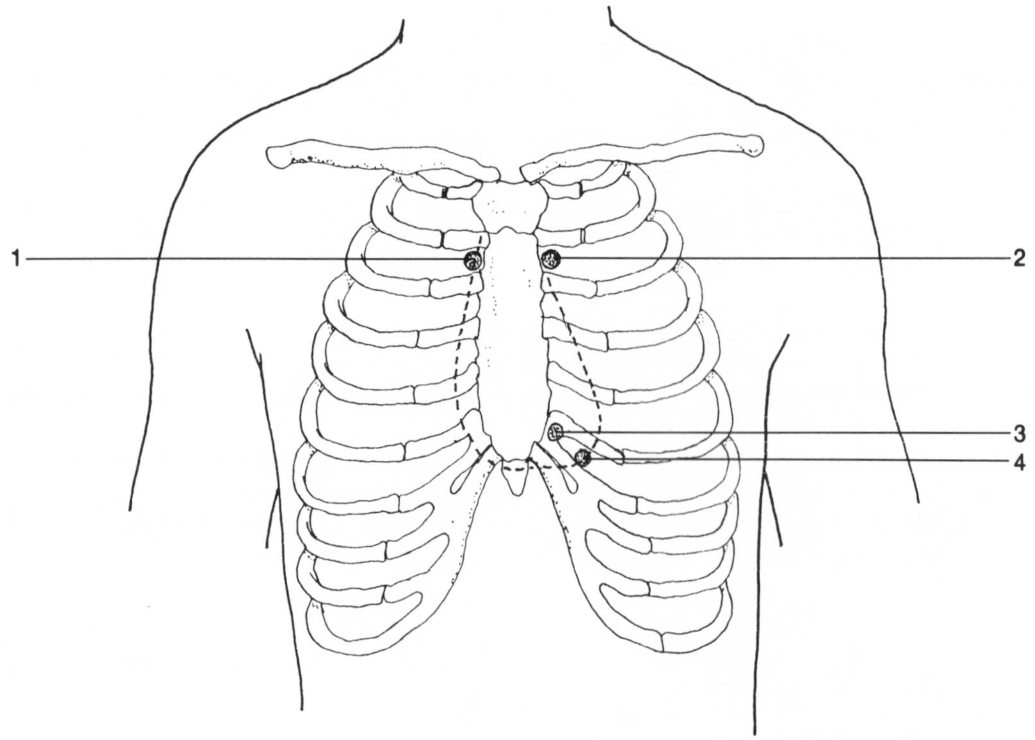

1
2
3
4

Label areas that describe the relation of heart sounds to the chest wall.

CHECK LIST
Cardiovascular System: Auscultation

Sex______________
Age______________

	Comments
Blood pressure method: palpation auscultation indicate *L.* (lying) *St.* (standing) R. arm	
L. arm	
R. thigh	
L. thigh	
pulse pressure	
Are your measurements within normal limits?	
If not, can you suggest possibilities for abnormal findings?	
Cardiac auscultation Identify the first and second heart sounds (S_1 and S_2), starting at the aortic or pulmonic area.	
Identify the heart rate (beats/min.). Is it within normal limits?	
Identify the rhythm (regular or irregular). If irregular, try to identify a pattern and describe it in writing.	
Listen at each of the seven auscultatory areas of the heart, first with the bell and then with the diaphragm. (Develop a systematic pattern.)	
At each area: Concentrate on the first heart sound; note its intensity, splitting.	
Concentrate on the second heart sound; note its intensity, splitting.	

	Comments
Listen for extra sounds in systole; note their timing, intensity, pitch.	
Listen for extra sounds in diastole; note their timing, intensity, pitch.	
Listen for systolic murmurs.	
Listen for diastolic murmurs. *If murmurs are present note the following characteristics:* timing	
location	
radiation or transmission (neck, sternal border, axilla)	
intensity (Grade I–VI)	
pitch	
quality	
Listen for murmurs or other cardiovascular sounds with both systolic and diastolic components.	

Examination should be performed in each of the five positions for complete cardiac evaluation. What effect does respiration have on various heart sounds?

Definitions

Match the definitions in *Column I* with the correct words in *Column II*.

Part I

____1 high arterial blood pressure
____2 subnormal arterial blood pressure
____3 the double sound caused by the slightly asynchronous closing of two heart valves
____4 a normal arrhythmia associated with respirations; the heartbeat becomes faster during inspiration and slower during expiration

A splitting
B hypertension
C sinus arrhythmia
D hypotension

Part II

____1 an abnormal auscultatory sound caused by blood going through a constricted vessel
____2 a grating sound produced by the rubbing together of inflamed or roughened surfaces
____3 a silent interval sometimes perceived during the determination of the blood pressure at a point some millimeters below the systolic pressure; failure to raise the cuff pressure high enough may give a false idea of systolic pressure if the phenomenon is present
____4 a triple cadence of the heart sounds at rates of 100 beats per minute or more due to an abnormal third or fourth heart sound that is heard in addition to the first and second sounds; usually indicative of serious cardiac disease
____5 fine, rapid, quivering movements of cardiac muscle that replace the normal myocardial contraction
____6 a murmur or soft sound (such as that made by a somewhat forcible expiration with the mouth open) heard on auscultation of the heart that is not caused by or indicative of organic heart disease
____7 murmur caused by a pathological condition

A innocent murmur
B friction rub
C organic murmur
D fibrillation
E bruit
F gallop rhythm
G auscultatory gap

Review Questions

Pediatric

1 What technique uses only a blood pressure cuff to obtain blood pressure in infants too small for auscultatory technique? Outline the steps you would take in utilizing this method.

2 Until what age would you expect the systolic blood pressure in the thigh to be equal to that in the arms?

3 A child with a venous hum in his neck should be referred. (true; false)

4 What can you have an eleven-year-old child do to help you decide if his arrhythmia is a sinus arrhythmia?

Adult

5 The pulse pressure is __________ mm Hg in a normal adult.

Both

6 The difference between the systolic and diastolic blood pressure is the __________.

7 Five factors that have a continuous influence on arterial pressure are:
1.
2.
3.
4.
5.

8 Because of its proximity to the heart, palpation of the __________ pulse is useful in timing cardiac events.

9 The blood pressure cuff size should not be more than __________ or less than __________ the length of the upper arm.

10 The minimum number of sounds that should be recorded when taking an arterial blood pressure is __________.

11 Difference in blood pressure taken from both arms of the same patient may vary up to __________ mm Hg. Difference greater than this suggests arterial compression or obstruction.

12 The normal pulse pressure expected throughout childhood is __________ mm Hg.

13 Biological factors that alter blood pressure include:
1.
2.
3.
4.
5.
6.
7.
8.

14 The three sounds recorded when measuring blood pressure by auscultation are identified by:
1.
2.
3.

15 List five positions the patient should assume during a complete cardiac exam.

16 The bell of the stethoscope is designed to pick up __________ and the diaphragm __________.

17 S_1 is generally louder than S_2 in which area?

18 S_2 is generally louder than S_1 in which area?

19 The carotid pulse is synchronous with (S_1; S_2).

20 Two things that may cause an increase in the intensity of S_1 are:
1.
2.

21 A split of S_2 is best heard __________.

22 A normal split of S_2 is widest with (inspiration; expiration).

23 A normal split of S_2 changes with position and respiration. (true; false)

24 A split that is unchanged by respiration is called __________.

25 Diagram normal heart sounds S_1 and S_2.

26 Diagram 3rd heart sound.

27 Diagram 4th heart sound.

28 In which area of auscultation is S_4 most likely to be heard?

29 During what phase of the cardiac cycle are you likely to hear S_4?

30 S_4 is most likely to be heard in an abnormal heart. (true; false)

31 Mediastinal crunch is most commonly heard following __________. Would you refer the patient for further evaluation?

32 Three abnormal sounds that can be detected by auscultation of the heart are:
1.
2.
3.

33 A split of S_2 is best heard at the __________ valve.

34 An abnormal splitting of S_1 would be heard at the __________.

35 All murmurs should be evaluated carefully and recorded with regard to:
1.
2.
3.
4.
5.
6.

36 Four characteristics of murmurs which mean that they are more likely to be innocent are:
1.
2.
3.
4.

Self-Evaluation Key

FIGURE 8–1 (p. 110, see p. 136)

FIGURE 8–2 (p. 111, see p. 137)

1. Label the cardiac chambers, valves and vessels.

11 left atrium
14 left ventricle
5 right atrium
15 right ventricle

13 aortic valve
12 mitral valve
6 pulmonary valve
7 tricuspid valve

8 aorta
4 inferior vena cava
9 left pulmonary artery
2 right pulmonary artery
16 main pulmonary artery
3, 10 pulmonary vein
1 superior vena cava

DEFINITIONS—BASIC KNOWLEDGE (pp. 112, 113)

1. D
2. G
3. A
4. J
5. M
6. Q
7. O
8. S
9. F
10. T
11. B
12. I
13. N
14. R
15. P
16. L
17. K
18. H
19. E
20. C

REVIEW QUESTIONS—BASIC KNOWLEDGE (p. 113)

PART I

1. SA node; AV node; bundle of His; Purkinje fibers
2. systole; rise
3. diastole; falls
4. mitral
5. aortic

PART II

1. rheumatic fever; CHD
2. rapid ventricular filling
3. atrial contraction
4. dyspnea; orthopnea; frequent URI's
5. cough; orthopnea; paroxysmal nocturnal dyspnea; cyanosis; noisy respirations
6. ascites; edema; fatigability

FIGURE 8–3 (p. 115)

1. sternoclavicular area
2. aortic area
3. pulmonic area
4. anterior precordium area
5. ectopic area
6. apical area (mitral area)
7. epigastric area

DEFINITIONS—INSPECTION (pp. 117, 118)

PART I

1. C
2. F
3. G
4. I
5. E
6. A
7. B
8. H
9. D
10. J

PART II

1. D
2. B
3. G
4. J
5. E
6. A
7. H
8. L
9. K
10. I
11. F
12. C

REVIEW QUESTIONS—INSPECTION (p. 118)

1. true (in children)
2. 4th or 5th left interspace, on or within the midclavicular line
3. true
4. false
5. tangential
6. expiration
7. an enlarged heart
8. ascites
9. scoliosis
10. cardiac enlargement
11. ventricular aneurysm

DEFINITIONS—PALPATION (p. 121)

PART I

1. C
2. A
3. B

PART II

1. B
2. D
3. A
4. C

REVIEW QUESTIONS—PALPATION (p. 122)

1. 4th or 5th; midclavicular
2. true
3. simultaneous auscultation of the heart or palpation of the carotid artery
4. abnormal
5. less
6. 1) left ventricular contraction
   2) blood volume
   3) capacity of the right heart to receive blood
7. sternal angle
8. Bates (Pressures and pulses: arterial and venous—anatomy and physiology)
9. 1) rate and rhythm
   2) amplitude
   3) contour
10. 1. carotid
    2. brachial
    3. femoral
    4. popliteal
    5. dorsalis pedis
    6. radial
    7. posterior tibial
11. fever; excitement; hyperthyroidism; severe anemia; cardiac disease
12. yes
13. true
14. true
15. stenosis of a valve; defect in the ventricular septum
16. location; transmission; timing in the cardiac cycle
17. abnormality
18. simultaneous auscultation of the heart or palpation of the carotid artery
19. radial; femoral

FIGURE 8–4 (p. 123, see p. 138)

REVIEW QUESTIONS—PERCUSSION (p. 125)

1. size; position or location
2. cardiac enlargement
3. a triangular area with one side of the triangle extending along the right sternal border from the 2nd to the 5th rib—the hypotenuse being the line from the right sternal border at the second rib to the midclavicular line of the 5th rib. (The heart of a young child is in a more horizontal position and the apex of the left border dullness is closer to the left nipple line than in the adult.)

FIGURE 8–5 (p. 126)

1. aortic area
2. pulmonic area
3. tricuspid area
4. mitral area

DEFINITIONS—AUSCULTATION (p. 129)

PART I

1. B
2. D
3. A
4. C

PART II

1. E
2. B
3. G
4. F
5. D
6. A
7. C

REVIEW QUESTIONS—AUSCULTATION (pp. 130, 131)

1. Flush Method/Flush Technique:
   a) place a suitable cuff on the wrist or ankle
   b) elevate the extremity
   c) compress distal portion of extremity by wrapping with an elastic bandage
   d) when compression is complete, lower extremity to heart level; rapidly inflate cuff to 200 mm Hg
   e) remove bandage and lower manometer pressure gradually at a rate of 5 mm Hg/sec
   f) at end point of determination, there will be the appearance of a "flush" in the extremity distal to the cuff.
2. 1 year
3. false
4. have him hold his breath
5. 30–50 mm Hg
6. pulse pressure
7. 1) cardiac output
   2) elasticity of arteries
   3) peripheral resistance
   4) blood volume
   5) blood viscosity
8. carotid
9. ⅔; ½
10. 3
11. 10 mm Hg
12. 20–50 mm Hg
13. 1) anxiety
    2) pain
    3) exertion
    4) eating of meals
    5) tobacco
    6) bladder distention
    7) climate variation
    8) emotional turmoil
14. 1) onset of muffling
    2) when sound becomes inaudible
    3) point at which the initial sound is heard for at least 2 consecutive beats.
15. 1) standing
    2) sitting straight
    3) lying flat on back
    4) sitting with chest bent forward
    5) lying on his left side
16. low frequencies, higher frequencies
17. apical
18. pulmonic or base
19. S_1
20. anemia; fever; exercise; tachycardia
21. pulmonic area
22. inspiration
23. true
24. fixed

25. see diagram below
26. see diagram below
27. see diagram below
28. at the apex
29. end of diastole
30. true
31. thoracic surgery; yes
32. S_4; pericardial friction rub; fixed split; paradoxical split; organic murmurs; ejection sounds; opening snap
33. pulmonic
34. apex
35. timing; location; radiation; intensity; pitch; quality
36. usually systolic; grade I or II; short duration; no transmission; don't affect growth and development; located in the pulmonic area

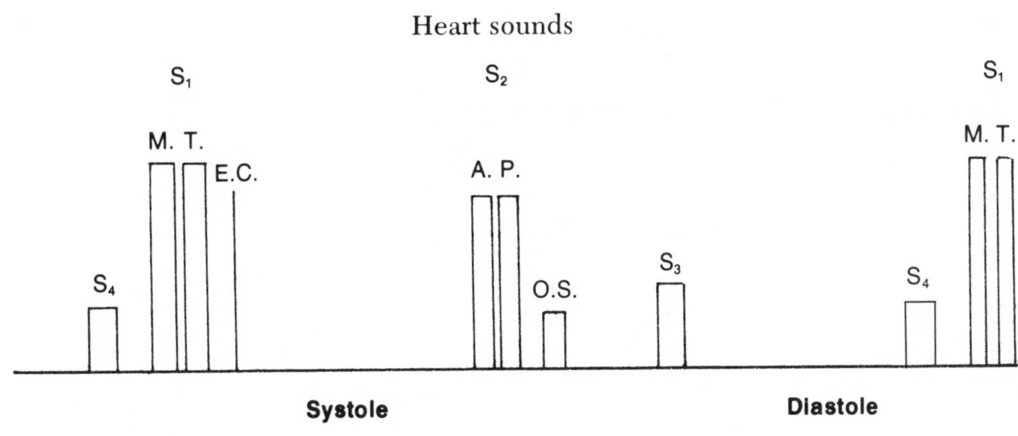

Self-Evaluation Key

Figure 8–1

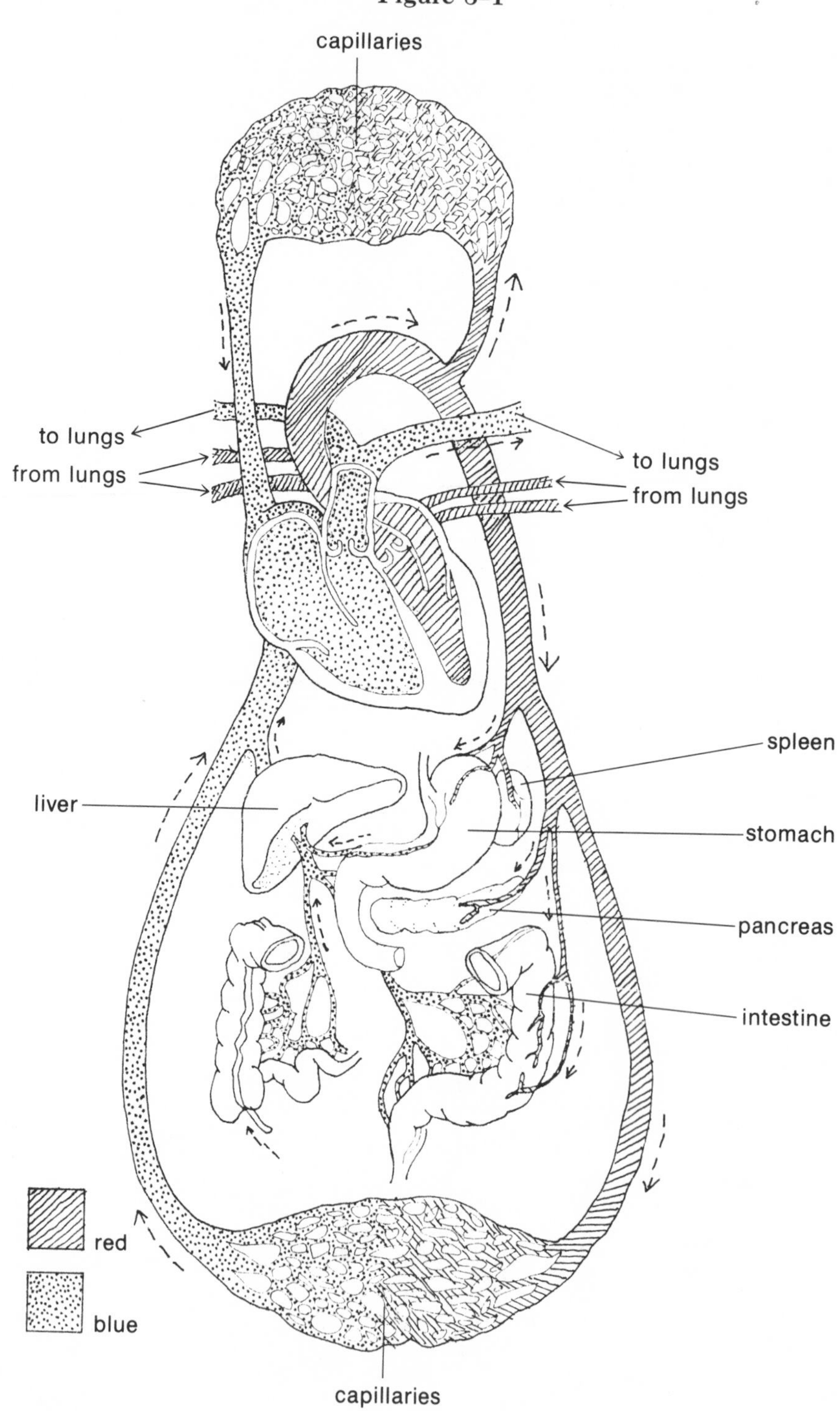

Figure 8–2

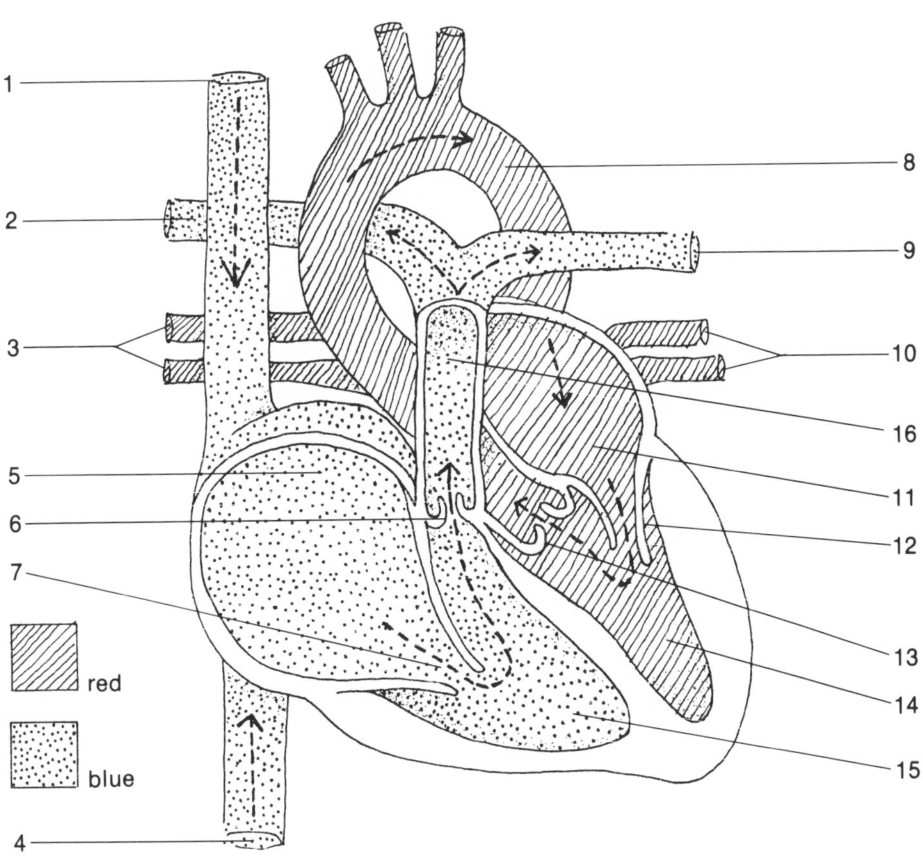

1. Label the cardiac chambers, valves and vessels.

11 left atrium

14 left ventricle

5 right atrium

15 right ventricle

13 aortic valve

12 mitral valve

6 pulmonary valve

7 tricuspid valve

8 aorta

4 inferior vena cava

9 left pulmonary artery

2 right pulmonary artery

16 main pulmonary artery

3,10 pulmonary vein

1 superior vena cava

Figure 8–4

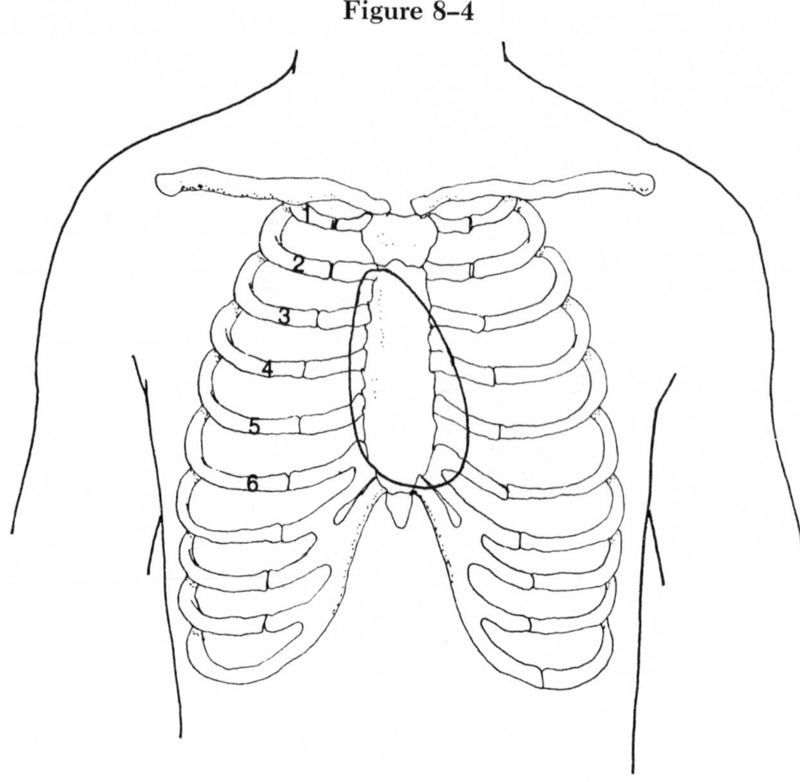

9

the breast

TO THE STUDENT

This section includes physical examination of the breast during pregnancy.

Recommended materials:

1 Alexander, Mary, and Brown, Marie. *Pediatric Physical Diagnosis for Nurses.* New York: McGraw-Hill Book Co., 1974

2 Bates, Barbara. *A Guide to Physical Examination,* Philadelphia: J. B. Lippincott Co., 1974

3 Blue Hill Educational Systems, Inc. *Physical Assessment Examinations—Breast* (Videotape: 15 minutes)

4 J. B. Lippincott Co. *Visual Guide to Physical Examination—Breasts* (Film/videotape: 7 minutes)

5 model of breast

6 access to three adult females and three children who will allow you to examine their breasts.

BASIC KNOWLEDGE

Behavioral Objectives

The student will be able to:

1 label the four quadrants of the breast on Figure 9–1

2 label the anatomical structures of the breast outlined on Figure 9–2

3 answer in writing all *Review Questions*

4 describe in writing the appropriate patient positions for examination of the breasts

5 state in writing the appropriate explanation for teaching a patient breast self-examination

6 answer in writing the optimal time, during a given month, to examine the breasts of a prepubertal child, menstruating woman, postmenopausal woman.

Learning Activities

I Required

A *Read:* Alexander and Brown; Bates

B *Label:* Figures 9–1 and 9–2

II Optional

See listing of additional references and materials specific to the breast.

Figure 9–1
Breast: quadrants*

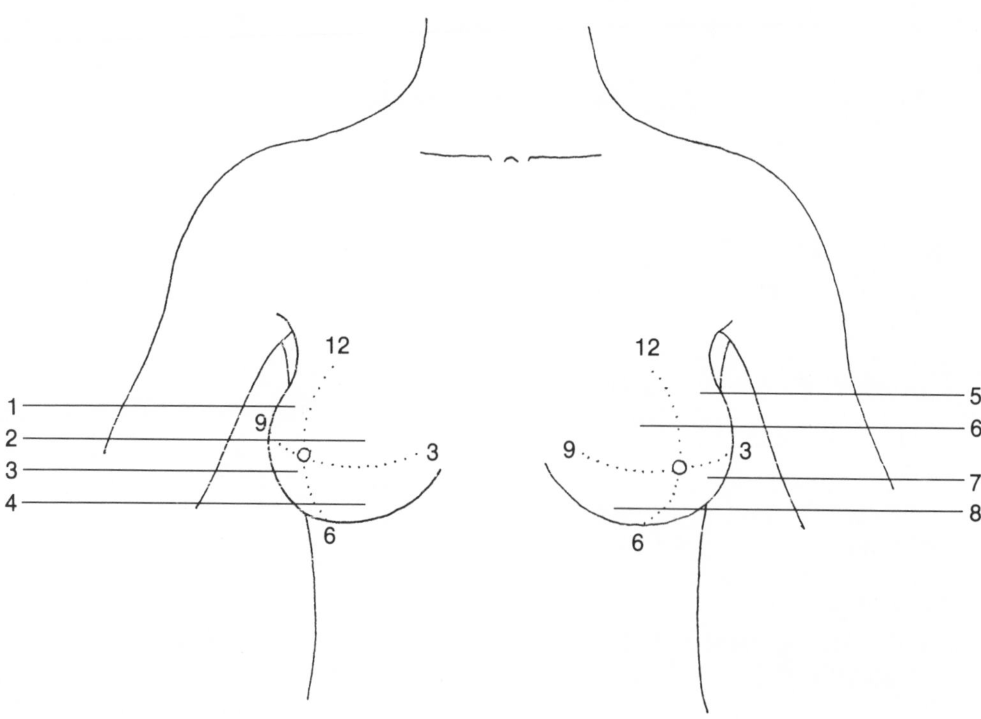

Label the four quadrants of the breast according to *Bates*.

1.
2.
3.
4.
5.
6.
7.
8.

*Note that each breast can also be considered as if it were the face of a clock with the nipple as the central point. Lesions can be located according to the axis of the clock in which they occur.

Figure 9–2
Breast

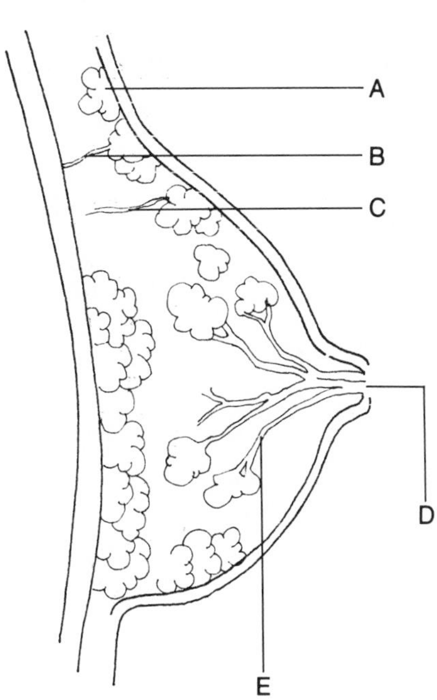

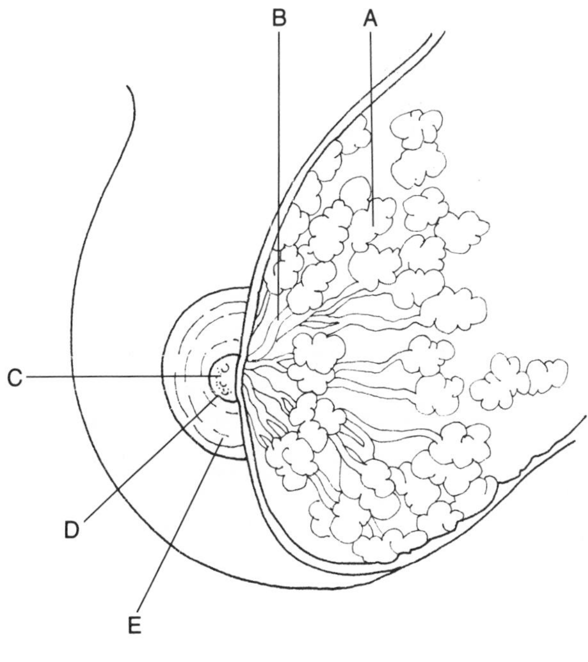

I

Label the following structures on *I*:

___ 1. fat

___ 2. glandular tissue

___ 3. duct

___ 4. opening of duct on nipple

___ 5. suspensory ligament

II

Label the following structures on *II*:

___ 1. opening of duct on nipple

___ 2. areola

___ 3. duct

___ 4. glandular tissue

___ 5. nipple

Review Questions

True—False

___1 The complete breast examination is performed with the patient in the recumbent position.

___2 It is seldom necessary to examine breast tissue in the male.

___3 Examination of the axillary nodes is performed as part of the breast examination.

___4 Menstruating women should routinely examine their breasts each month at the *end* of the menstrual period.

___5 The breasts sometimes engorge premenstrually and during pregnancy.

INSPECTION

Behavioral Objectives

The student will be able to:

1 state that inspection of the breast includes observation of the skin, symmetry, size, contour, venous pattern, and presence of discharge
2 state in writing the differences (found on inspection) between the breasts of a pregnant woman and the breasts of a nonpregnant woman
3 state which observations are within normal limits and which warrant further investigation
4 define in writing the terms listed under *Definitions*
5 answer in writing all *Review Questions*
6 describe and record appropriately on the check list provided the physical findings related to inspection of the breasts of three children and three adult females.

Learning Activities

Required

A *Read:* Alexander and Brown; Bates
B *View:* Blue Hill Series videotape *Physical Assessment—Breast*
C Examine and record findings on inspection of the breasts of three adult females and three children, using the check list provided.

CHECK LIST
Breast: Inspection

The following list should be filled in for each inspection required in the learning activities.

Sex__________ **Pregnant**__________ **Lactating**__________
Age__________ **Prepubertal**__________
Menstruating__________
Menopausal__________

Observations	Yes	No	Describe Variations or Abnormalities
skin: rash			
normal color (breast tissue and areola)			
venous pattern			
scars			
edema/thickening			
lesions			
striae			
symmetrical			
size abnormality			
contour: masses			
dimpling			
flattening/retraction			
nipple inverted			
nipple everted			
discharge			

Definitions

Match the definitions in *Column I* with the correct words in *Column II*.

____1 circular pigmented area surrounding the nipple, or papilla mammae
____2 inflammation of the breast; most common in the female during lactation, but it may occur at any age; breast has a nodular feeling on palpation
____3 excessive development of the male mammary glands; milk is sometimes secreted
____4 accessory nipple
____5 a shrinking, drawing back; state of being drawn back
____6 a turning inward

A retraction
B mastitis
C areola
D inversion
E supernumerary nipple
F gynecomastia

Review Questions

TRUE—FALSE

Adult:
____1 Dimpling of the skin sometimes suggests an underlying malignancy.
____2 During pregnancy the nipple color darkens.
Adult and Pediatric:
____3 Simple nipple inversion of long standing is a common normal variant.
____4 The presence of nipple discharge usually implies an underlying malignancy.
____5 Nonbloody nipple discharge does not require further evaluation.

SELECTION

6 Check the physical findings below that warrant referral or further investigation:
____a. recent development of inversion in a previously erect nipple
____b. left breast slightly larger than right
____c. nipple deviation
____d. unilateral nipple drainage
____e. unilateral dilated superficial veins

7 Describe the appropriate procedures for inspecting the breasts. (Include patient position and maneuvers.)

PALPATION

Behavioral Objectives

The student will be able to:

1 state how to demonstrate a systematic method for palpating the breast
2 state that palpation of the breast includes noting the presence of warmth, tenderness, masses, nodules in the breasts and in the axillary lymph nodes
3 state which findings are within normal limits and which require further investigation
4 state that masses must be described according to size, contour/discreteness, consistency, mobility, location, and tenderness
5 answer in writing all *Review Questions*
6 describe and record appropriately on the check list provided the physical findings related to palpation of the breasts of three children and three adult women.

Learning Activities

Required

A *Read:* Alexander and Brown; Bates
B *View:* Blue Hill Series videotape *Physical Assessment—Breast*
C *Work with model* of breast
D *Examine and record findings* on palpation of the breasts of three adult females and three children, using check list provided.

CHECK LIST

Breast: Palpation

The following list should be filled in for each examination (palpation) required in the learning activities:

Sex________ **Prepubertal**________ **Lactating**________
Age________ **Menstruating**________
Menopausal________
Pregnant________

Observations	Yes	No	Describe Variations or Abnormalities
Breast tissue normal consistency/elasticity			
tenderness			
heat			
masses *describe:* size			
discreteness/contour			
consistency			
mobility			
location			
tenderness			
nipples masses			
discharge expressed			
lymph nodes *include:* lateral axillary group			
central group			
pectoral group			
describe: heat			
tenderness			
enlargement			
mobility			
location			

Review Questions

TRUE—FALSE

Adult and Pediatric

____1 During palpation, breast tissue is compressed against the pectoralis major muscle.

____2 The principles for examination of the male breast differ from those for the female breast.

____3 Carcinoma of the breast is usually apparent earlier in men than in women.

SELECTION

4 Check the physical findings below that warrant referral or further investigation:

____a. bilateral premenstrual fullness and tenderness
____b. warm, tender, enlarged axillary node
____c. tender, palpable nodules in the (R) areola
____d. multiple tender nodules (bilateral)
____e. solitary, firm, nontender nodule in upper outer quadrant of (L) breast

5 The most frequent site of breast malignancy is in the:

____a. upper outer quadrant
____b. lower inner quadrant
____c. upper inner quadrant

Self-Evaluation Key

FIGURE 9–1 (p. 140)

1. upper outer
2. upper inner
3. lower outer
4. lower inner
5. upper outer
6. upper inner
7. lower outer
8. lower inner

FIGURE 9–2 (p. 141)

PART I

1. A
2. C
3. E
4. D
5. B

PART II

1. C
2. E
3. B
4. A
5. D

REVIEW QUESTIONS—BASIC KNOWLEDGE (p. 141)

1. F
2. F
3. T
4. T
5. T

DEFINITIONS—INSPECTION (p. 144)

1. C
2. B
3. F
4. E
5. A
6. D

REVIEW QUESTIONS—INSPECTION (p. 144)

1. T
2. T
3. T
4. F
5. F
6. a, c, d, e
7. See Bates, pp. 148–150

REVIEW QUESTIONS—PALPATION (p. 147)

1. T
2. F
3. T
4. b, c, d, e
5. a

10

the abdomen

TO THE STUDENT

Because of the special requirements of the abdominal examination, auscultation precedes percussion and palpation in this section. It should be noted that examination of the pregnant abdomen is included in this section, as is examination of the rectum. Palpation for femoral pulses is covered in the section on the cardiovascular system (Section 8).

Recommended materials:

1 Alexander, Mary, and Brown, Marie. *Pediatric Physical Diagnosis for Nurses.* New York: McGraw-Hill Book Co., 1974
2 Bates, Barbara. *A Guide to Physical Examination.* Philadelphia: J. B. Lippincott Co., 1974
3 "Patient Assessment—Examination of the Abdomen." Programmed Instruction. *American Journal of Nursing* 74(September 1974): 1679–1702
4 Blue Hill Educational Systems, Inc. *Pediatric Physical Examination—The Abdomen & Genitalia* (Videotape: 44 minutes)
5 Blue Hill Educational Systems, Inc. *Physical Assessment Examinations—Abdomen* (Videotape: 35 minutes)
6 Ciba Pharmaceutical Co. *Examination of the Abdomen: Pediatric.* (Film)
7 J. B. Lippincott Co. *Visual Guide to Physical Examination—Abdomen* (Film/videotape: 9 minutes)
8 access to three adults and three children who will allow you to examine their abdomens

BASIC KNOWLEDGE

Behavioral Objectives

The student will be able to:

1 answer in writing all *Review Questions*

2 label the major anatomical landmarks on Figure 10–1
3 label the epigastric area and periumbilical area, on Figure 10–1
4 draw in and label the abdominal quadrants and the major anatomical structures located in each abdominal quadrant, as listed in Figure 10–2
5 describe in writing the appropriate patient position for examination of the abdomen and rectum
6 state in writing the appropriate order of the examination methods used in examination of the abdomen.

Learning Activities

I Required
A *Read:*
Alexander and Brown; Bates
AJN programmed instruction "Patient Assessment—Examination of the Abdomen," pp. 1679–1702
B *View:*
1 Blue Hill Series videotapes *Pediatric Examination—The Abdomen & Genitalia; Physical Assessment—Abdomen*
2 Ciba film *Examination of Abdomen: Pediatric*
C *Label:* Figure 10–1
D *Draw:* The designated structures in Figure 10–2
II Optional
See listing of additional references and materials specific to the abdomen in *Bibliography*.

Figure 10–1
Abdomen: epigastric and periumbilical areas

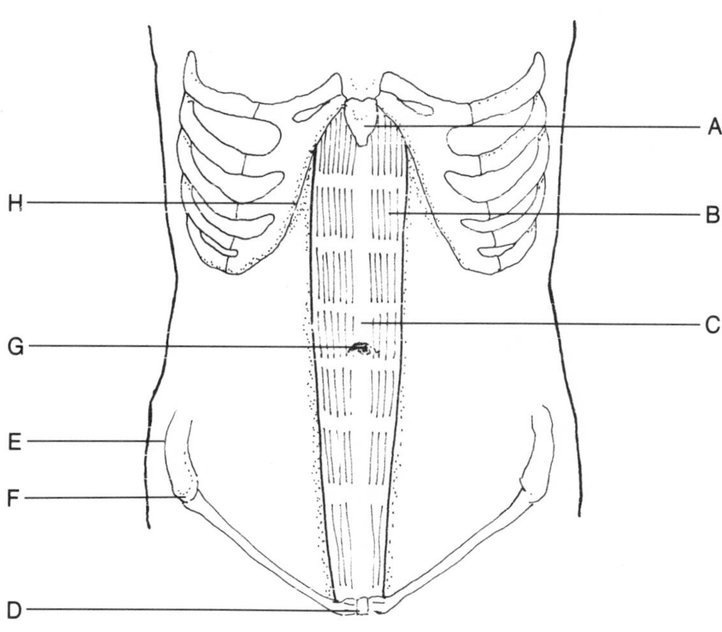

Directions:

1. Draw in the epigastric and periumbilical areas
2. Label:

___ 1. costal margin

___ 2. umbilicus

___ 3. iliac crest

___ 4. anterior superior iliac spine

___ 5. rectus abdominis muscle

___ 6. xiphoid process

___ 7. symphysis pubis

___ 8. midline

Figure 10–2
Abdominal quadrants

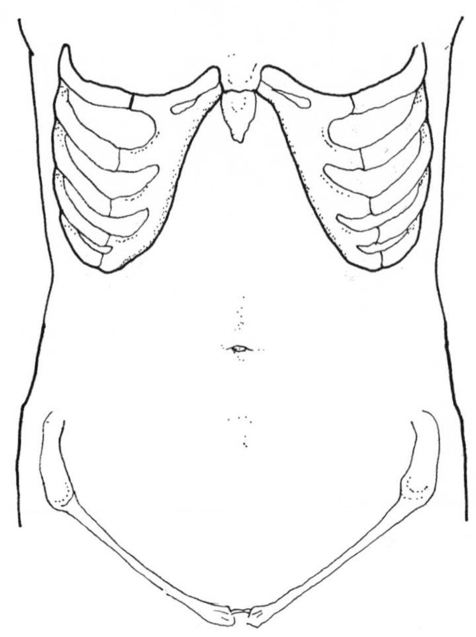

Directions:

1. Draw in the four abdominal quadrants.
2. Draw and label the following structures in the appropriate location on the diagram above:

a. liver
b. stomach
c. spleen
d. cecum
e. sigmoid colon
f. pancreas
g. duodenum
h. left ovary and tube
i. right ovary and tube
j. right kidney
k. hepatic flexure of colon
l. left kidney
m. splenic flexure of colon
n. appendix
o. gallbladder
p. bladder
q. uterus
r. abdominal aorta

Review Questions

True—False

____1 In examination of the abdomen, palpation is performed first.

____2 The *right* quadrants are separated from the *left* quadrants by a line that extends vertically from the xiphoid to the symphysis pubis.

____3 The patient should be placed in a supine position for examination of the abdomen.

____4 The anal canal is liberally supplied by somatic sensory nerves, making this examination potentially painful.

Matching

5 (Match the following structures with the quadrant in which they are normally located. Some questions may have more than one correct answer.)

____1 cecum
____2 pancreas
____3 sigmoid colon
____4 splenic flexure of colon
____5 left kidney
____6 right ovary and tube
____7 duodenum
____8 spleen
____9 appendix
____10 uterus
____11 liver
____12 stomach
____13 left ovary and tube
____14 right kidney
____15 hepatic flexure of colon
____16 gallbladder
____17 bladder
____18 abdominal aorta

A right upper
B left upper
C right lower
D left lower

INSPECTION

Behavioral Objectives

The student will be able to:

1 define in writing the terms listed under *Definitions*

2 answer in writing all *Review Questions*

3 state that inspection of the abdomen includes observation of skin, contour of the abdominal wall, superficial blood vessels, respiratory movements, peristaltic movements, hair distribution, and the umbilicus

4 state that inspection of the anal area includes observation for evidence of skin lesions, external hemorrhoids, fissures, fistulas, rashes, inflammation, or lumps

5 describe and record appropriately on the check list provided the physical findings related to inspection of the abdomens of three adults and three children of varying ages.

Learning Activities

I Required

A *Read:*

1 Alexander and Brown

2 Bates

3 *AJN* programmed instruction "Patient Assessment—Examination of the Abdomen," pp. 1679–1702

B *View:*

1 Blue Hill Series videotapes *Pediatric Examination—The Abdomen & Genitalia; Physical Assessment—Abdomen*

2 Ciba film *Examination of Abdomen: Pediatric*

C *Examine and record findings:* inspection of the abdomens of three adults and three children of varying ages. (Use check list provided.)

II Optional

See listing of additional references and materials specific to the abdomen.

CHECK LIST

The Abdomen: Inspection

The following list should be filled in for each inspection required in the learning activities.

Sex_____________
Age_____________

	Yes	No	Describe (*where appropriate*)
Skin			
rashes			
lesions			
color normal for this patient			
striae			
scars			
glistening, thick skin			
drainage from umbilicus			
Pigmentation			
jaundice			
bluish discoloration of umbilicus			
bluish discoloration of flanks			
Contour			
symmetry of contour			
symmetrically protuberant			
symmetrically scaphoid			
umbilicus centrally located			
lower abdominal fullness			
bulging flanks			
Umbilicus			
umbilicus deeply inverted			
umbilicus flat or everted			
visible umbilical hernia			
Movement			
visible peristaltic waves			
visible respiratory movement			
aortic pulsations			
fetal movements			
Vessels			
distended abdominal veins			
direction of blood flow is away from umbilicus (if abdominal veins are distended)			
cutaneous angiomas (spider nevi)			
Hair distribution			
pubic hair in shape of triangle, with base above symphysis pubis			
pubic hair in shape of diamond			
generalized abdominal hair distribution			
curly pubic hair			
straight pubic hair			
presence of pubic lice			

Definitions

Match the definitions in *Column I* with the correct words in *Column II.*

Part I

____1 boat shaped; hollowed; abdomen may have this appearance in starvation or malnutrition

____2 a stripe, band, streak, or line distinguished by color, texture, depression, or elevation from the tissue in which it is found; may be due to overstretching of the skin, as in pregnancy or ascites

____3 enlargement of an organ (e.g., *hepatomegaly* means "enlargement of the liver")

____4 rupture; the protrusion of an organ or part of an organ or other structures through the wall of the cavity normally containing it

____5 a maneuver in physical examination to estimate the size of an organ not near the surface, particularly when there is ascites, by a flicking motion of the hand or fingers similar to that of dribbling a basketball; applied particularly to a method of diagnosis of pregnancy —with the tip of the forefinger in the vagina a sharp tap is made against the lower segment of the uterus; the embryo, if present, is tossed upward, and if the finger is retained in place will presently be felt to strike against the wall of the uterus as it falls back; used to test for engagement of the fetal head

A organomegaly

B ballottement

C scaphoid

D hernia

E stria

Part II

____1 an accumulation of serous fluid in the peritoneal cavity

____2 an arteriole angioma in the skin, seen most commonly in hepatic disease, but occasionally during pregnancy; has a central red body that may be raised above the skin level and several radiating branching legs that run parallel to and just beneath the skin surface; also called spider nevus

____3 congenital eventration at the umbilicus

____4 a crack or slit in the mucous membrane of the anus; very painful and very difficult to heal

A omphalocele

B ascites

C anal fissure

D cutaneous angioma

Review Questions

True—False

Adult

____1 A fine, visible venous network may normally be present in an adult.
____2 Peristalsis may be visible normally in very thin adults.
____3 Spider nevi are associated with liver disease.

Pediatric

____4 Peristalsis is normally seen in children.
____5 In a crying infant, a bulge between the recti muscles is always abnormal.
____6 An infant normally has a more protuberant abdomen than an adult.
____7 Excessive protuberance of the pediatric abdomen may indicate starvation.

Both

____8 A normal aortic pulsation is frequently visible in the epigastrium.
____9 The abdomen normally retracts at the beginning of inspiration.
____10 A generalized scaphoid abdomen could indicate malnutrition.
____11 A bluish discoloration of the flanks, in the presence of trauma, may be indicative of intra-abdominal hemorrhage.

Completion

Pediatric

12 Reversed peristaltic waves in the infant are often associated with __________.

Adult

13 Tight, glistening skin is often associated with __________.
14 Striae are usually associated with __________.

Both

15 An increase in visible peristaltic waves is associated with __________.
16 Describe the normal direction of blood flow in the abdominal veins.

17 Describe how the examiner can determine the direction of blood flow in the distended veins of the abdomen.

AUSCULTATION

Behavioral Objectives

The student will be able to:

1 answer in writing all *Review Questions*
2 distinguish between normal and abnormal bowel sounds when listening to an abdomen
3 recognize the sounds of skin and hair on the stethoscope as differentiated from other findings on auscultation
4 recognize the normal sounds of the stomach
5 distinguish fetal heart sounds from the maternal aortic pulse*
6 state which auscultatory findings are within normal limits and which ones would warrant referral to a physician
7 describe and record appropriately on the check list provided the physical findings related to auscultation of the abdomens of three adults and three children.

Learning Activities

Required

A *Read:*
 1 Alexander and Brown
 2 Bates
 3 *AJN* programmed instruction "Patient Assessment—Examination of the Abdomen," pp. 1670–1702

B *View:*
 1 Blue Hill Series videotapes *Pediatric Examination—The Abdomen & Genitalia; Physical Assessment—Abdomen*
 2 Ciba film *Examination of Abdomen: Pediatric*

C *Examine and record findings* of your auscultation of the abdomens of three adults and three children of varying ages.

*This is not covered in the readings. It is done simply by palpating the mother's pulse while at the same time auscultating the fetal heart. If the two are synchronous, the mother's heart is being auscultated. If they are asynchronous, fetal heart tones are being auscultated.

CHECK LIST

Abdomen: Auscultation

The following list should be filled in for each auscultation required in the learning activities.

Sex______________
Age______________

Peristalsis	**Yes**	**No**	**Describe** (*where appropriate*)
peristalsis present in RUQ			
LUQ			
RLQ			
LLQ			
frequency within normal limits			
character within normal limits			

PERCUSSION

Behavioral Objectives

The student will be able to:

1 answer in writing all *Review Questions*
2 state a systematic approach to percussion of the abdomen
3 identify by percussion the upper and lower borders of liver dullness in the midclavicular line during both inspiration and expiration
4 state that any dullness extending above the ninth interspace in the left midaxillary line indicates enlargement of a solid organ
5 state that the mean diameter of liver dullness is about 10 cm
6 state which findings on percussion are within normal limits and which would warrant referral to a physician
7 describe and record appropriately on the check list provided the physical findings related to percussion of the abdomens of three adults and three children
8 identify ascites by the maneuvers of:
  a) fluid wave
  b) shifting dullness.

Learning Activities

Required

A *Read:*
  1 Alexander and Brown
  2 Bates
  3 *AJN* programmed instruction "Patient Assessment—Examination of the Abdomen," pp. 1679–1702

B *View:*
  1 Blue Hill Series videotapes *Pediatric Examination—The Abdomen & Genitalia; Physical Assessment—Abdomen*
  2 Ciba film *Examination of Abdomen: Pediatric*

C *Examine and record findings* on percussion of the abdomens of three adults and three children of varying ages.

CHECK LIST
Abdomen: Percussion

The following list should be filled in for each percussion required in the learning activities.

Sex__________
Age__________

	Yes	No	Describe (*where appropriate*)
Liver upper limit of liver dullness in midaxillary line from 5th to 7th interspace (note if during inspiration or expiration)			
lower limit of liver dullness at costal margin (note if during inspiration or expiration)			
mean diameter of liver dullness 10–12 cm (in adult)			
Stomach tympany in the area of the left lower anterior rib cage			
Spleen resonant in lowest interspace in L anterior axillary line			
Abnormal fluid presence of fluid wave			
shifting dullness			

Review Questions

1 Describe where the examiner would stand and the order he would follow in percussing the abdomen.

2 Describe the technique for detecting ascites by the fluid wave.

3 Describe the technique for detecting ascites by shifting dullness.

COMPLETION
(Fill in the blanks)

4 The normal upper limit of liver dullness in the midaxillary line varies from the ________ to the ________ interspace.
5 The lower border of liver dullness is at the ________.
6 Most of the abdomen sounds ________ to percussion.
7 If the urinary bladder is distended, the examiner will note ________ to percussion.
8 The percussion note during inspiration in the lowest intercostal space in the left anterior axillary line should be ________, provided the spleen is not enlarged.

PALPATION

Behavioral Objectives

The student will be able to:

1 answer in writing all *Review Questions*
2 describe in writing the procedure of palpation in terms of positioning the patient and assisting him to become relaxed
3 state in writing that the description of any mass should include size, shape, location, pulsation, consistency, contour, mobility, and tenderness
4 state in writing how to perform each of the Leopold maneuvers on a pregnant abdomen and describe the purpose of each maneuver
5 assess tissue turgor of the abdomen
6 state in centimeters the expected distance from the symphysis pubis to the uterus during each week from the twelfth to the thirty-sixth week of pregnancy
7 palpate correctly for rebound tenderness
8 palpate correctly for enlargement of intra-abdominal organs: spleen, liver, and kidneys
9 palpate correctly for masses
10 palpate the umbilicus for any masses or hernias
11 palpate for femoral and ventral hernias
12 palpate for diastasis recti
13 state in writing the correct method of palpation for inguinal hernias
14 state in writing the correct method for palpation of the anus and rectum for the presence or absence of stricture; for tone of anal sphincter, thrombosed internal hemorroids, tumors, or polyps; for size, shape, and consistency of prostate
15 describe and record appropriately on the check list provided the physical findings related to palpation of the abdomens of three adults and three children.

Learning Activities

Required

A *Read:*
  1 Alexander and Brown
  2 Bates
  3 Danforth, pp. 265–267
  4 *AJN* programmed instruction "Patient Assessment—Examination of the Abdomen," pp. 1679–1702

B *View:*
  1 Blue Hill Series videotapes *Pediatric Examination—The Abdomen & Genitalia; Physical Assessment—Abdomen*
  2 Ciba film *Examination of Abdomen: Pediatric*

C *Examine and record findings* from palpation of the abdomens of three adults and three children of varying ages.

CHECK LIST

The Abdomen: Palpation

The following list should be filled in for each palpation required in the learning activities.

Sex____________
Age____________

	Yes	No	Describe (*where appropriate*)
Presence of pain/tenderness			
Masses on light palpation			
on deep palpation			
Organ enlargement kidney right			
left			
spleen			
liver			
Palpable aorta			
Tissue turgor normal			
Muscle tone increased			
normal tonus			
flaccid			
uterus			
Femoral hernia right			
left			
Diastasis recti			
Inguinal hernia right			
left			
Subcutaneous crepitus			

TO THE STUDENT: In most respects, the physical examination of the pregnant female is very similar to that of the nonpregnant person. There are some very specific maneuvers related to palpation of the pregnant abdomen, however. Because the textbooks on physical assessment do not discuss these maneuvers, you will not find them in your assigned readings. Therefore they will be discussed here and will be highlighted in the *Review Questions*.

Measurement of Fundal Height

Measurement of fundal height is important because it is an indication of how far along a pregnancy has progressed. Although there are several other methods of determining the due date of a pregnancy, measurement of fundal height is a very important one (Figure 10–3). If this measurement does not agree with the calculations derived from the other methods (for instance, counting from the last menstrual period or dating from the time when fetal heart tones are first heard), it may be a warning sign (1) that the other dates are inaccurate, or (2) that for some reason the uterus is growing at a faster or slower rate than is normal. This might happen, for instance, with twins (in which case it would grow faster) or with certain anomalies that make a baby smaller than expected (in which case it would grow more slowly).

These measurements are taken by holding one end of a tape measure at the symphysis pubis and stretching the other end until it reaches the fundus of the uterus, which can be palpated as a very firm, rounded organ. There are three measurements to keep in mind:

1 the fundus can first be palpated *just above the symphysis pubis at 10 weeks of gestation*
2 it can be felt *halfway between the symphysis and the umbilicus at 16 weeks*
3 it can be felt *at the umbilicus at 20 weeks.*

These measurements are called "Spiegelberg's Measurements." Some other measurements expected according to this calculation are:

Linear distance, symphysis to fundus (cm)	Estimated fetal age (weeks)
26.7	28
30.0	32
32.0	36

After 36 weeks, these measurements become inaccurate because of the limited room in the abdomen.

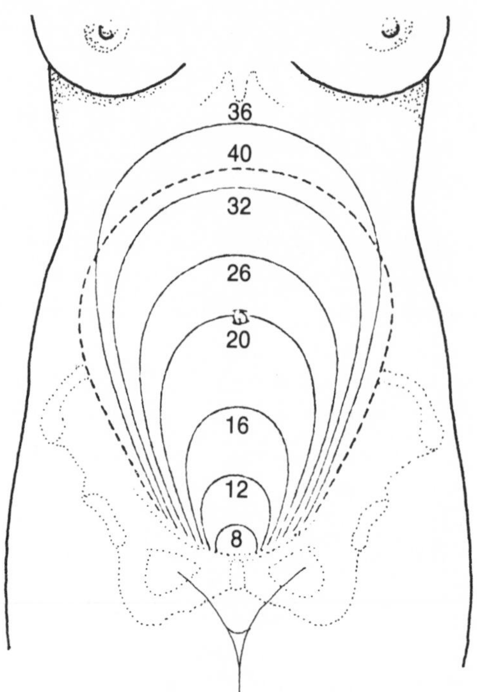

Figure 10–3
Height of fundus

Height of fundus at comparable gestational dates shows great variation from patient to patient. Those shown above are perhaps most frequent. Convenient rule of thumb is that at 5 months gestation, fundus is usually at or slightly above umbilicus. (From David N. Danforth, *Textbook of Obstetrics and Gynecology*, 2nd ed. Figure by Douglas M. Haynes, M.D. Copyright 1971, Harper & Row Publishers, Inc.)

Leopold Maneuvers

Another important method of palpating the uterus is known as the *Leopold maneuvers.* This is a method of determining the position of the fetus that is useful in the latter months of pregnancy and occasionally during labor. The four maneuvers are:

1. *Fundal palpation*

In this maneuver, the examiner stands at the woman's feet looking toward her head. The fingertips of both hands gently outline the fetal part that occupies the fundus. In a normal pregnancy this will be the fetal head, which should feel firm and round. In a breech presentation the buttocks will be palpated; in this presentation, the examiner will feel a softer, less firm, more nodular sensation.

2. *Palpation for spine and extremities*

The next maneuver is performed with the examiner standing in the same position. This time the examiner's hands are placed on each side of the uterus. On one side will be a hard, firm, long structure—the back; on the other side will be a series of nodular parts—the extremities. In an obese abdomen, the hard, firm back may be the only palpable part.

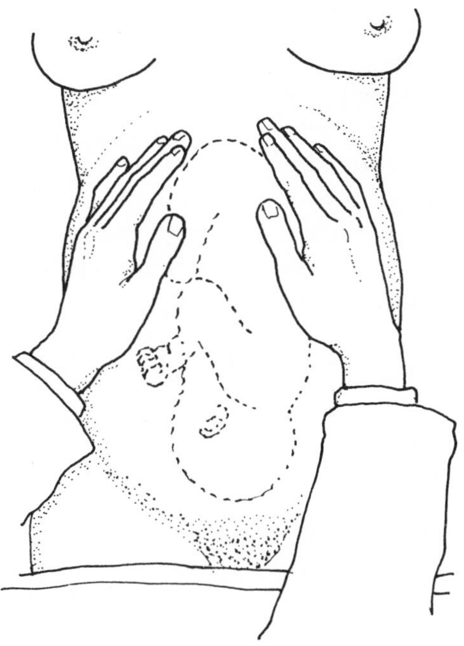

Figure 10–4
Fundal palpation

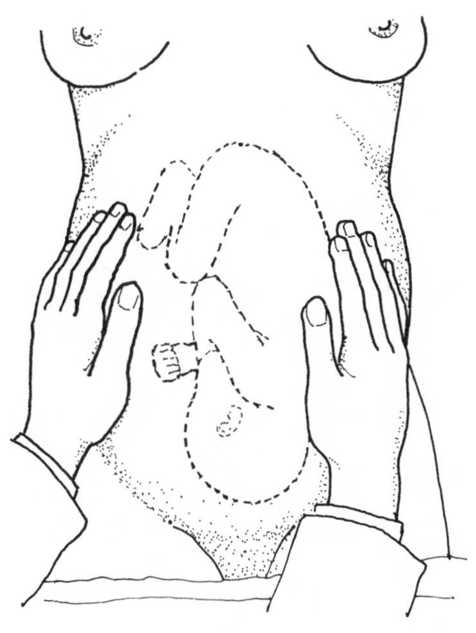

Figure 10–5
Palpation for spine and extremities

3. *Palpation of presenting part*

The examiner remains in the same position for the third maneuver. This time the part of the uterus directly above the symphysis pubis is palpated by grasping it firmly between the thumb and fingers of one hand. As in the first maneuver, the examiner begins by differentiating between the hard, firm roundness of the head and the softer, more nodular consistency of the buttocks. Occasionally (for instance, in a footling presentation) an extremity will be palpated. In a cephalic presentation, the very skilled examiner can differentiate between a fetus whose neck is flexed and one whose neck is extended. In a cephalic presentation, the examiner then tries to determine if the fetus is engaged by pushing upward on the head. If it is not yet engaged, a ballotable sensation will result.

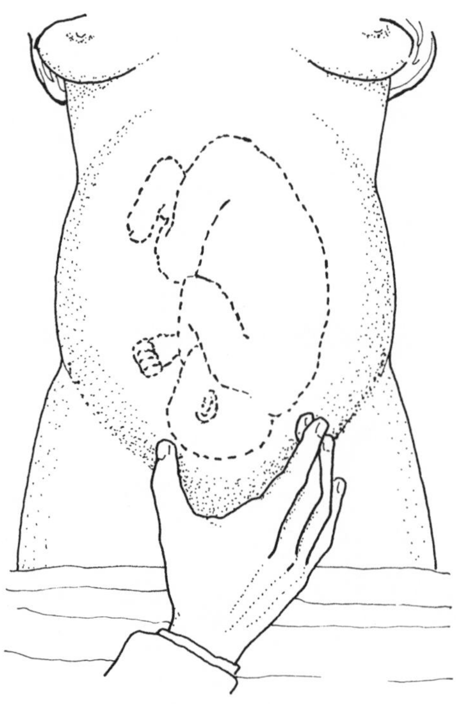

Figure 10–6
Palpation of the presenting part

4. *Further palpation of the presenting part*

For the last maneuver, the examiner remains on the same side of the woman, but turns to face her feet rather than her head. In this position, the examiner exerts gentle, firm, deep pressure with the middle three fingers of each hand in a downward direction, pushing under the symphysis pubis. Again an evaluation is made of whether the presenting part is a head or buttocks; and again an attempt is made to decide whether the head is flexed or extended. The depth of the presenting part indicates how far engagement has progressed; in a baby who is completely engaged, it may be impossible to feel the head, and only the soft shoulder can be palpated.

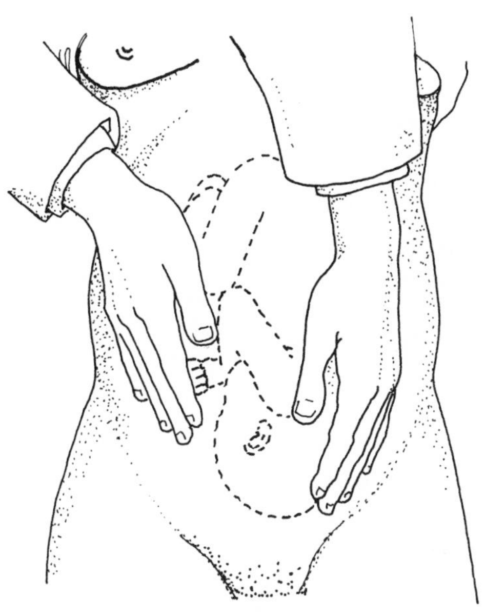

Figure 10–7
Further palpation of the presenting part

Review Questions

True—False

Pediatric

______ 1 A liver that is palpable 3 cm below the costal margin in a three year old is always abnormal.

______ 2 A palpable spleen tip is always abnormal in an infant.

Adult

______ 3 The prostate gland should be small, symmetrical, nonmovable, and have a rubbery consistency.

______ 4 Any palpation of the prostate in the rectal lumen is indicative of enlargement.

______ 5 The spleen is normally palpable in the adult.

______ 6 The cecum may be palpable in thin adults.

______ 7 The liver is normally palpable at 6 cm below the costal margin in the adult.

______ 8 In chronic emphysema the liver is less likely to be palpable.

______ 9 Internal hemorrhoids cannot be felt unless thrombosis is present.

______ 10 A hard, stony area on the prostate may indicate carcinoma.

Both

______ 11 The examiner should use light palpation before using deep palpation.

______ 12 During deep palpation in the midepigastrium, almost all patients will complain of tenderness, which accompanies pressure on the abdominal aorta.

______ 13 The spleen normally moves down with inspiration.

______ 14 The gallbladder is normally palpable.

______ 15 In the rectal examination of the female, the cervix presents as a small, round mass in the anterior wall.

______ 16 Having the patient bear down during the rectal examination makes a tumor palpable that would otherwise be inaccessible.

______ 17 Pain caused by inflammation usually remains unchanged or increases as pressure is applied.

______ 18 Visceral pain caused by distention tends to become more severe while pressure is maintained.

______ 19 Discomfort from intra-abdominal sources will be less severe when the abdomen is tense than when it is relaxed, due to muscle guarding.

______ 20 Rebound tenderness is found only when the peritoneum overlying a diseased viscus becomes inflamed.

______ 21 When the patient lifts his head from the examining table, abdominal wall masses will remain palpable.

______ 22 Femoral hernias are seen as soft masses that protrude into the anterior abdominal wall.

______ 23 Umbilical hernias are congenital in origin and are best seen when the patient coughs or strains.

______ 24 An inguinal hernia may contain either bowel or mesentery.

______ 25 The external inguinal rings are examined for inguinal hernias.

Pregnant

______ 26 The second Leopold maneuver is used to ascertain which pole of the fetus lies in the fundus.

______ 27 The third Leopold maneuver indicates that the lower pole of the fetus is fixed in the pelvis.

Multiple Choice

28 According to Spiegelberg's Measurements, you would expect a pregnant uterus to reach the umbilicus at
- a. 10 weeks
- b. 16 weeks
- c. 20 weeks
- d. 24 weeks

29 Leopold's maneuvers are
- a. methods of determining gestational age
- b. methods of ballottement of an enlarged spleen
- c. methods of palpating an enlarged liver
- d. methods of determining fetal presentation

30 You would expect to find that the uterine fundus of a 16 week gestation was
- a. not yet palpable
- b. palpable halfway between the symphysis pubis and the umbilicus
- c. barely palpable above the symphysis pubis
- d. palpable at the umbilicus

Self-Evaluation Key

FIGURE 10–1 (p. 151)

1. H
2. G
3. F
4. E
5. B
6. A
7. D
8. C

See Bates for areas drawn in.

FIGURE 10–2 (p. 152)

See anatomy text.

REVIEW QUESTIONS—BASIC KNOWLEDGE (p. 153)

1. F
2. T
3. T
4. T
5. 1. C
   2. A and B
   3. D
   4. B
   5. B
   6. C
   7. A
   8. B
   9. C
   10. C and D
   11. A
   12. B
   13. D
   14. A
   15. A
   16. A
   17. C and D
   18. A and B

DEFINITIONS—INSPECTION (p. 156)

PART I

1. C
2. E
3. A
4. D
5. B

PART II

1. B
2. D
3. A
4. C

REVIEW QUESTIONS—INSPECTION (p. 157)

1. T	5. F	9. F
2. T	6. T	10. T
3. T	7. T	11. T
4. F	8. T	

12. pyloric stenosis
13. ascites
14. weight gain/weight loss
15. intestinal obstruction
16. away from umbilicus
17. A segment of vein in the epigastrium is emptied between two fingers to a distance of a few cms. One then allows blood to refill the vein from one direction by removing one finger and observing rate of filling. Same segment is again emptied, and filling from opposite direction is estimated. Usually rate of flow is obviously faster in one direction—thus indicating direction of flow.

REVIEW QUESTIONS—PERCUSSION (p. 162)

1. stand on patient's right: *1st*—down L thoracic wall in midaxillary line
   2nd—percuss down R side in midaxillary line and keep liver span
   3rd—remainder of abdomen
2. See Bates
3. See Bates
4. 5th to 7th
5. costal margin
6. tympanitic
7. dullness
8. resonant

REVIEW QUESTIONS—PALPATION (p. 170)

1. F	9. T	17. T	24. T
2. F	10. T	18. F	25. T
3. F	11. T	19. T	26. F
4. T	12. T	20. T	27. T
5. F	13. T	21. T	28. c
6. T	14. F	22. F	29. d
7. F	15. T	23. T	30. b
8. F	16. T		

11

male genitalia

TO THE STUDENT

Recommended materials:

1 Alexander, Mary, and Brown, Marie. *Pediatric Physical Diagnosis for Nurses.* New York: McGraw-Hill Book Co., 1974

2 Bates, Barbara. *A Guide to Physical Examination.* Philadelphia: J. B. Lippincott Co., 1974

3 Blue Hill Educational Systems, Inc. *Pediatric Physical Examination—The Abdomen & Genitalia* (Videotape: 44 minutes)

4 Blue Hill Educational Systems, Inc. *Physical Assessment Examinations—Genito-Urologic* (Videotape: 12 minutes)

5 J. B. Lippincott Co. *Visual Guide to Physical Examination—Male Genitalia* (Film/videotape: 10 minutes)

6 male genitalia model

7 two male children, an infant and a child under one year, on whom you will examine the genitalia.

BASIC KNOWLEDGE

Behavioral Objectives

The student will be able to:

1 answer in writing all *Review Questions*

2 define in writing the terms listed under *Definitions*

3 label a diagram illustrating the pertinent anatomical structures of the male genitalia.

Learning Activities

I Required
  A *Read:* Alexander and Brown; Bates
  B *Label:* Figure 11–1
II Optional
  See listing of additional references and materials specific to genitalia in *Bibliography*.

Figure 11–1
Male genitalia

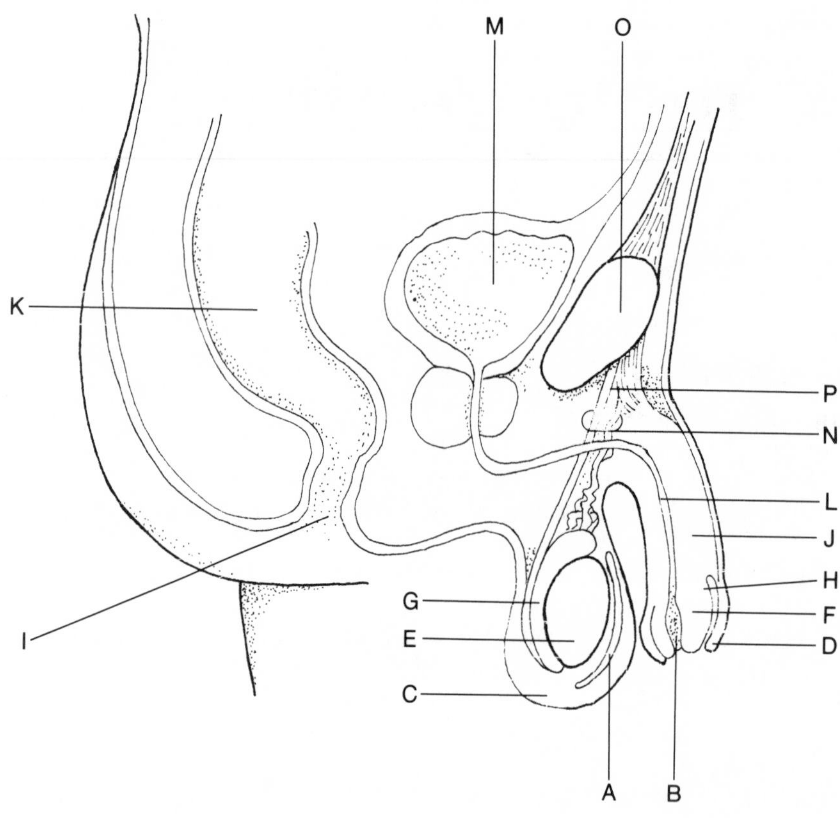

Label:

___ 1. scrotum	___ 9. prepuce
___ 2. epididymis	___ 10. pubis
___ 3. anus	___ 11. glans
___ 4. vas deferens	___ 12. corona
___ 5. urethra	___ 13. testis
___ 6. rectum	___ 14. tunica vaginalis
___ 7. bladder	___ 15. spermatic cord
___ 8. urethral meatus	___ 16. shaft of penis

Definitions

Match the definitions in *Column I* with the correct words in *Column II*.

Column I

____**1** principal portion of the penis; the cylindrical body of the penis

____**2** foreskin; the free fold of skin that more or less completely covers the glans penis

____**3** the conical expansion of the corpus spongiosum, which forms the head of the penis

____**4** the prominent posterior border of the glans penis

____**5** a musculocutaneous sac containing the testis

____**6** one of the two male reproductive glands, located in the cavity of the scrotum

____**7** the secretory duct of the testicle, running from the epididymis, of which it is the continuation, to the prostatic urethra, where it terminates as the ejaculatory duct

____**8** one of two folded, sacculated, glandular structures, each of which is a diverticulum of the vas deferens; its secretion is one of the components of semen

____**9** the duct formed by the union of the vas deferens and the excretory duct of the seminal vesicle, which opens into the prostatic urethra

____**10** a chestnut-shaped body, partly muscular and partly glandular, which surrounds the beginning of the urethra in the male; it secretes a milky fluid that is discharged into the urethra at the time of emission of semen, mixing with this secretion

____**11** the cord formed by the vas deferens and its associated structures, extending from the deep inguinal ring through the inguinal canal into the scrotum

____**12** the first convoluted portion of the excretory duct of the testis; passes from above, downward along the posterior borders of this gland; at the lower extremity of the testis it turns upward and gradually merges into the vas deferens

____**13** drawing up of the scrotum and testicles of the same side when the skin on the inner side of the thigh is scratched

Column II

A spermatic cord
B prostate
C cremasteric reflex
D epididymis
E shaft
F glans
G ejaculatory ducts
H prepuce
I corona (corona glandis)
J seminal vesicle
K scrotum
L vas deferens
M testicle

Review Questions

TRUE—FALSE

Pediatric

____1 Urethral and genital abnormalities are associated with a high incidence of other birth defects.

____2 In the smaller child, the testes should be examined at the beginning of the exam to prevent stimulating withdrawal into the abdomen.

Both

____3 Normally, the urethra is located dorsally in the shaft of the penis.

____4 Phimosis refers to a tight foreskin.

____5 The testes descend along the femoral canal into the scrotum.

____6 Normally, compression of the testes is painful.

____7 Torsion of the spermatic cord requires *immediate* treatment.

INSPECTION AND PALPATION

Behavioral Objectives

The student will be able to:

1 answer in writing all *Review Questions*

2 define in writing the terms listed under *Definitions*

3 describe in writing a systematic approach to performing this examination

4 label a diagram illustrating the course and presentation of inguinal and femoral hernias in the groin

5 perform an examination of the genitalia of two male children (an infant and a child under one year) and record findings appropriately on the check list provided.

Learning Activities

Required

A *Read:* Alexander and Brown; Bates

B *Label:* Figure 11–2

C *View:* Blue Hill Series videotapes *Pediatric Examination—The Abdomen & Genitalia; Physical Assessment—Genito-Urologic*

D *Examine:*

1 a model of the male genitalia, including an examination of the prostate gland

2 two males (an infant and a child under one year) and record findings on the check list provided.

Figure 11-2

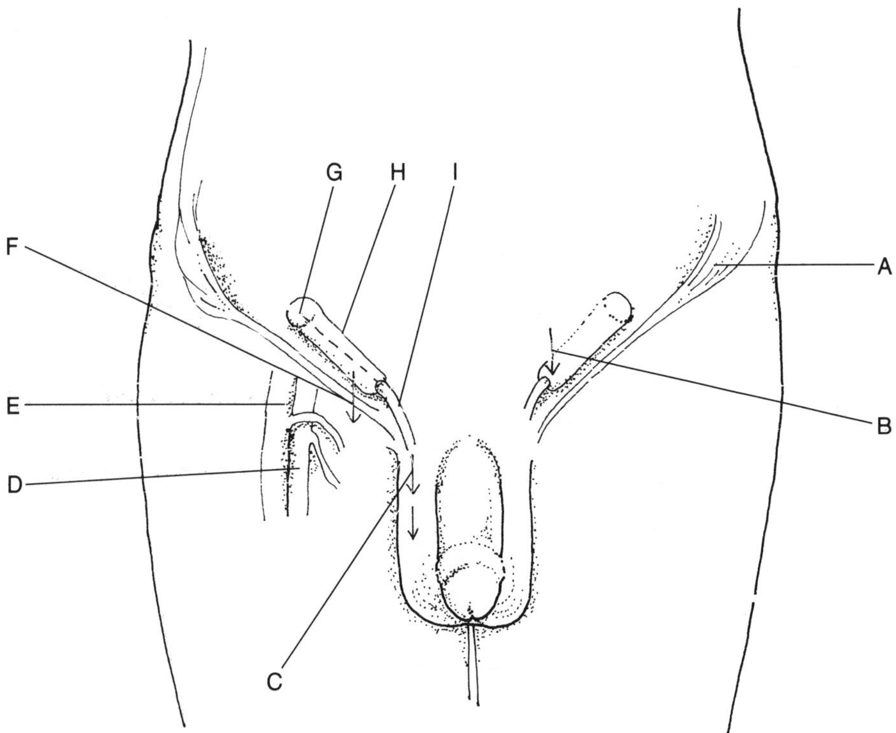

Label:

1. external inguinal ring
2. inguinal canal
3. femoral vein
4. femoral artery
5. internal inguinal ring
6. course of direct inguinal hernia
7. course of indirect inguinal hernia
8. course of femoral hernia
9. inguinal ligament

CHECK LIST
Inspection and Palpation

Age______________

	Yes	No	Describe (*where appropriate*)
Hair distribution			
Penis skin normal color			
lesions			
foreskin present			
retractable			
lesions			
glans lesions			
nodules			
urethral meatus normal position			
discharge			
inflammation			
size atrophic			
enlarged			
normal for age			
Scrotum skin normal color			
lesions			
rugae			
Testes size			
shape			
consistency			
tenderness			
location			
number palpable			
Inguinal canal size			
bulges			

	Yes	No	Describe (*where appropriate*)
Epididymis			
size			
shape			
consistency			
tenderness			
location			
Spermatic cord/vas deferens			
swelling			
nodules			
Anus			
normal surrounding tissue			
lesions			
excoriation			
fissure			
lumps, nodules			
tenderness			
sphincter tone			
pilonidal cyst			
Rectum			
normal surface			
nodules			
masses			
hemorrhoids			
internal			
external			
prolapse			
fissure			
polyps			
Prostate gland			
size			
shape			
consistency			
tenderness			
nodules			

Definitions

Match the definitions in *Column I* with the correct words in *Column II.*

_____1 a developmental anomaly characterized by a defect in the wall of the urethra, so that the canal is open for a greater or lesser distance on the under surface of the penis

_____2 a malformation of the penis in which the urethra opens on the upper surface

_____3 a collection of serous fluid in a sacculated cavity such as the testis

_____4 inflammation of the glans penis

_____5 narrowness of the opening of the prepuce (foreskin), which prevents its being drawn back over the glans

_____6 inflammation of the urethra

_____7 primary lesion; the first manifestation of syphilis; it begins as a papule or area of infiltration, of dull red color, hard and insensitive; the center usually becomes eroded or breaks down into an ulcer

_____8 soft or simple chancre; an infectious venereal ulcer developing on an inflamed edematous base from a pustule

_____9 persistent erection of the penis, especially when due to disease and not sexual desire

_____10 constriction of the glans penis by a foreskin with a narrow orifice, which has been retracted behind the corona and cannot be drawn forward

_____11 inflammation of the epididymis

_____12 inflammation of the testis

_____13 a cystic, usually pyriform enlargement of the epididymis containing spermatozoa

_____14 a varicose enlargement of the veins of the spermatic cord, causing a boggy tumor of the scrotum

_____15 a swelling due to effusion of blood into the tunica vaginalis testis

A epididymitis
B hematocele
C spermatocele
D varicocele
E orchitis
F hypospadias
G paraphimosis
H balanitis
I epispadias
J priapism
K phimosis
L chancroid
M hydrocele
N chancre
O urethritis

Review Questions

True—False

Pediatric

____**1** All authorities agree that the foreskin should always be retracted as part of the examination of a child under four months of age.

Both

____**2** The left testis usually is somewhat lower than the right testis.
____**3** The testes are the most palpable structures in the scrotum.
____**4** Anteversion of the epididymis is a normal variant.
____**5** Scrotal swelling containing blood will transilluminate.
____**6** Scrotal edema is usually associated with generalized edema.

Multiple Choice

7 A generalized scrotal mass consisting of blood is a
a) spermatocele
b) hematocele
c) hydrocele

8 The condition in which the urinary meatus is located dorsally on the penis is called:
a) epispadias
b) hypospadias

Self-Evaluation Key

FIGURE 11–1 (p. 174)

1. C
2. G
3. I
4. P
5. L
6. K
7. M
8. B
9. D
10. O
11. F
12. H
13. E
14. A
15. N
16. J

DEFINITIONS—BASIC KNOWLEDGE (p. 175)

1. E
2. H
3. F
4. I
5. K
6. M
7. L
8. J
9. G
10. B
11. A
12. D
13. C

REVIEW QUESTIONS—BASIC KNOWLEDGE (p. 176)

1. T
2. T
3. F
4. T
5. F
6. T
7. T

FIGURE 11–2 (p. 177)

1. I
2. H
3. D
4. E
5. G
6. B
7. C
8. F
9. A

DEFINITIONS—INSPECTION AND PALPATION (p. 180)

1. F
2. I
3. M
4. H
5. K
6. O
7. N
8. L
9. J
10. G
11. A
12. E
13. C
14. D
15. B

REVIEW QUESTIONS—INSPECTION AND PALPATION (p. 181)

1. F
2. T
3. T
4. T
5. F
6. T
7. b
8. a

12

female genitalia

TO THE STUDENT

The section on the female genitalia includes bimanual, pelvic, and rectal examinations. Since inspection and palpation are closely related in these examinations, they will be considered together. Please note that the inguinal lymph nodes should be routinely examined as part of the external genitalia exam. This particular area, however, is covered in the section on the skin and lymphatic system (Section 2).

Recommended materials:

1 Alexander, Mary, and Brown, Marie. *Pediatric Diagnosis for Nurses.* New York: McGraw-Hill Book Co., 1974
2 Bates, Barbara. *A Guide to Physical Examination.* Philadelphia: J. B. Lippincott Co., 1974
3 Blue Hill Educational Systems, Inc. *Pediatric Physical Examination—The Abdomen & Genitalia* (Videotape: 10 minutes)
4 Blue Hill Educational Systems, Inc. *Physical Assessment Examinations—Gynecologic* (Videotape: 16 minutes) and *Genito-Urologic* (Videotape: 12 minutes)
5 J. B. Lippincott Co. *Visual Guide to Physical Examination—Female Genitalia* (Film/videotape: 10 minutes)
6 model of the female pelvis
7 two female children, an infant and a child under one year, in whom you will examine the genitalia

BASIC KNOWLEDGE

Behavioral Objectives

The student will be able to:

1 answer in writing all *Review Questions*
2 define in writing the terms listed under *Definitions*
3 label the anatomical structures of the female external genitalia as shown on Figure 12–1
4 label the anatomical structures of the vagina and cervix as shown on Figure 12–2
5 state in writing the effects of estrogen (or lack of estrogen) on the vulva, vagina, and cervix.

Learning Activities

I Required
A *Read:* Alexander and Brown; Bates
B *Label:* Figure 12–1 and Figure 12–2
II Optional
See listing of additional references and materials specific to genitalia in *Bibliography.*

Figure 12–1
Female genitalia: external structures

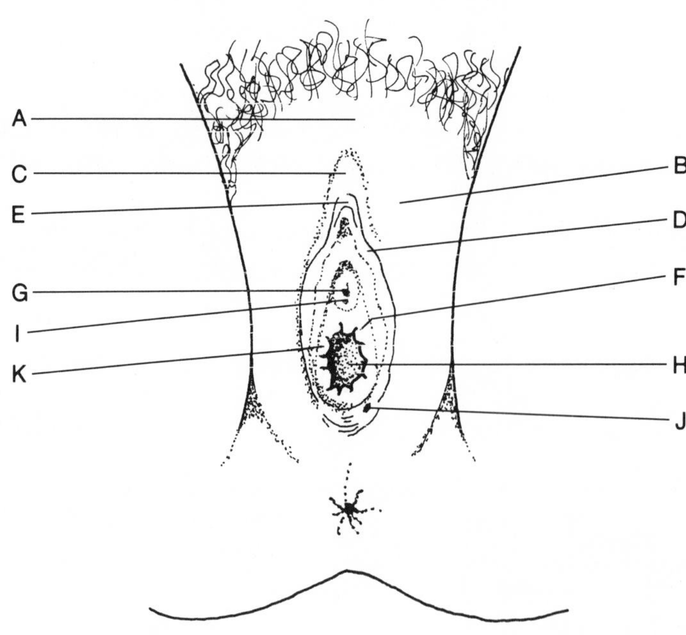

Label:

___ 1. opening of Bartholin's gland
___ 2. clitoris
___ 3. vagina
___ 4. mons veneris
___ 5. opening of Skene's gland
___ 6. labium minus (plural *labia minora*)*
___ 7. labium majus (plural *labia majora*)*
___ 8. vestibule
___ 9. prepuce
___ 10. urethral meatus
___ 11. hymen

*Labia are separated for visualization of structures between them.

Figure 12–2
Female genitalia: cross section

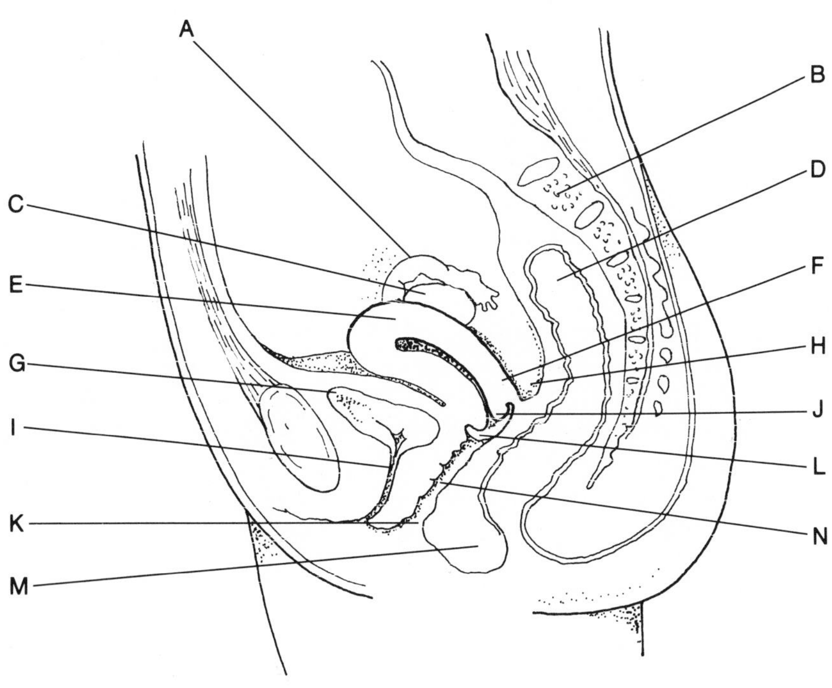

Label:

____ 1. perineum

____ 2. rectum

____ 3. vagina

____ 4. uterus

____ 5. isthmus of uterus

____ 6. bladder

____ 7. sacrum

____ 8. fallopian tube

____ 9. introitus

____ 10. urethra

____ 11. ovary

____ 12. rectouterine pouch

____ 13. anterior fornix

____ 14. cervix

Definitions

Match the definitions in *Column I* with the words in *Column II*.

____1 the triangular area of coarse pubic hair in the adult
____2 a small, cylindrical, erectile body, rarely exceeding 2 cm in length, situated at the most anterior portion of the vulva and projecting between the branched extremities of the labia minora; it is the analogue of the penis in the male except that it is not perforated by the urethra
____3 vulva; the external genital organs of the female
____4 entrance to the vagina; the space behind the glans clitoridis and between the labia minora, containing the openings of the vagina, urethra, and ducts of Bartholin's glands
____5 one of the numerous mucous glands in the wall of the female urethra
____6 a thin, membranous fold partly or wholly occluding the external orifice of the vagina
____7 two mucous glands on either side of the lower part of the vagina
____8 the external fold of the labia minora, forming a cap over the clitoris
____9 pubis or pubic region

A pudendum
B Skene's gland
C female escutcheon
D mons veneris
E clitoris
F Bartholin's glands
G vestibule (vaginae)
H hymen
I prepuce (clitoridis)

Review Questions

True—False

Adult and Pediatric
____1 Female escutcheon refers to a type of senile vaginitis.
____2 The inguinal lymph system drains the pelvic area.
____3 Lack of estrogen increases the friability of vaginal mucosa.
____4 For examination of the genitalia, a female patient should be in the dorsal recumbent position.
____5 The clitoris is composed of erectile tissue.
____6 The frenulum is a thin membrane covering part of the vaginal orifice.
____7 In the absence of estrogen, female genital structures atrophy.
Pediatric
____8 A vaginal examination is seldom performed on a prepubertal child.
____9 The vulva of an infant has more subcutaneous tissue than the vulva of a postmenopausal woman.

Multiple Choice

Pediatric
10 The *primary* reason for examining the genitalia of an infant is to
a. reassure the parents that the infant is normal
b. determine that the organs are intact
c. be certain that there is no ambiguity about the child's gender

Both
11 Name the external structures of the female genitalia.

INSPECTION AND PALPATION (INCLUDING BIMANUAL AND PELVIC EXAMINATIONS)

Behavioral Objectives

The student will be able to:

1 answer in writing all *Review Questions*
2 define in writing the terms listed under *Definitions*
3 describe and *demonstrate* a systematic approach for performing this examination
4 perform an examination of the female genitalia (on a model) including the speculum exam and bimanual exam; record findings appropriately according to the check list provided
5 describe cervical changes commonly seen in pregnancy
6 state in writing an appropriate method for obtaining a Pap smear.

Learning Activities

Required

A *Read:* Alexander and Brown; Bates
B *View:* Blue Hill Series videotapes *Pediatric Examination—The Abdomen & Genitalia; Physical Assessment—Gynecologic* and *Genito-Urologic**
C *Examine:*
  1 a model of the female pelvis; include the external genitalia, speculum exam of the vagina and cervix, and bimanual exam
  2 the genitalia of a female infant and record findings according to the check list provided.

*Students may wish to view additional films on the gynecologic examination; for instance, the OMNI Series *Gyn Exam* or the University of Washington film *The Female Pelvic Exam*.

CHECK LIST
Female Genitalia: Inspection and Palpation

The following list should be completed for each examination (including the examination of the model) required in the learning activities.

Age____________
Model____________

	Yes	No	**Describe** (*where appropriate*)
External genitalia			
hair distribution			
vulva			
lesions			
inflammation			
sores/warts			
rash			
discharge			
swelling			
clitoris normal for age			
vestibule			
Bartholin's glands visible			
urethra			
inflammation			
Skene's gland inflamed			
discharge			
stress incontinence			
vagina			
hymen intact			
discharge			
inflammation			
lesions			

	Yes	No	Describe (*where appropriate*)
Internal			
cervix			
color normal			
os (parous/nonparous)			
discharge			
size normal			
symmetrical			
position normal			
lesions			
IUD string visible			
erosion, eversion			
tender			
Pap smear done.			
uterus			
position normal			
size normal for age			
shape normal			
firm			
mobile			
tender			
masses			
ovaries			
size normal			
firm			
mobile			
tenderness of any palpable masses			
rectum			
nodules			
masses			
hemorrhoids			
prolapse			
fissure			
polyps			

Definitions

Match the definitions in *Column I* with the words in *Column II.*

Part I

_____1 dark bluish or purplish discoloration of the vaginal and cervical mucous membranes; a presumptive sign of pregnancy

_____2 the examination of a smear of body secretions, especially from the cervix or vagina, fixed immediately, while wet, in alcohol; the appearance of exfoliated cells in the smears may be used in the early detection of cancer or to evaluate the hormonal status of the patient

_____3 inflammation of the urethra

_____4 inflammation of the vulva

_____5 to fall or sink down; said of an organ or other part; a condition of the uterus when the cervix may present well beyond the vaginal orifice

_____6 leakage of urine as a result of coughing, straining, or some sudden voluntary movement; due to weakness of the muscles around the neck of the bladder and surrounding the vagina, resulting in an incompetent internal vesical sphincter

A prolapse

B urethritis

C Chadwick's sign

D stress incontinence

E Papanicolaou smear

F vulvitis

Part II

_____1 hernia of the bladder; downward displacement of the bladder towards the vaginal orifice

_____2 prolapse of the rectum forming a herniation through the posterior wall of the vagina

_____3 a projecting warty growth on the external genitals or at the anus consisting of fibrous overgrowths covered by thickened epithelium; usually produced by the irritating discharges in chronic vaginal infections

_____4 a wearing away; a state of being worn away

_____5 a turning outward

_____6 generic term for a large group of molds or fungi that are commonly known as "fruit molds." A few closely related, potentially pathogenic organisms formerly classified in this genus are now properly termed *Candida*

_____7 acute or subacute vaginitis or urethritis caused by infection with *Trichomonas vaginalis,* a flagellate; characterized by varying degrees of tenderness in the pelvis, hyperemia of the mucosa, moderate numbers of petechiae and a yellow or yellow-white, frothy, thin, putrid discharge that may lead to painful chafing of the vulva

_____8 an accumulation of mucus or other nonsanguineous fluid in the vagina

_____9 an accumulation of menstrual blood in the vagina because of imperforate hymen or other obstruction

_____10 a retention cyst that develops when a gland of the cervix uteri is obstructed as the result of its duct becoming plugged with squamous epithelium; the latter is formed from metaplasia of the normal epithelium during chronic inflammation of the cervix

A hydrocolpos

B *Monilia*

C cystocele

D nabothian cyst

E trichomoniasis

F rectocele

G hematocolpos

H eversion

I condyloma accuminatum

J erosion

Review Questions

TRUE—FALSE

Adult

____**1** Venous congestion in the cervix during pregnancy is referred to as "Hagar's sign."

____**2** The most accurate sample of cells for the Pap smear is obtained from the cervix and endocervical canal.

____**3** The vaginal speculum is most safely and comfortably inserted vertically.

____**4** The nulliparous os is small and round in shape.

Adult and Pediatric

____**5** Erosion of the cervix refers to the absence of covering epithelium.

____**6** *Monilia* vaginitis can always be determined by inspection.

____**7** Bulging of the bladder and anterior vaginal wall into the introitus is called a rectocele.

Adult

8 Describe the procedure for obtaining a Pap smear.

Both

9 Describe a systematic method for examining the external female genitalia.

Self-Evaluation Key

FIGURE 12–1 (p. 184)

1. J
2. E
3. H
4. A
5. I
6. D
7. B
8. K
9. C
10. G
11. F

FIGURE 12–2 (p. 185)

1. M
2. D
3. N
4. E
5. F
6. G
7. B
8. A, K
9. K
10. I
11. C
12. H
13. L
14. J

DEFINITIONS—BASIC KNOWLEDGE (p. 186)

1. C
2. E
3. A
4. G
5. B
6. H
7. F
8. I
9. D

REVIEW QUESTIONS—BASIC KNOWLEDGE (p. 186)

1. F
2. T
3. T
4. F
5. T
6. F
7. T
8. T
9. F
10. c
11. mons veneris, prepuce, clitoris, urethral meatus, opening of Skene's gland, vestibule, labia majora, labia minora, hymen, vagina, opening of Bartholin's gland

DEFINITIONS—INSPECTION AND PALPATION (p. 190)

PART I

1. C
2. E
3. B
4. F
5. A
6. D

PART II

1. C
2. F
3. I
4. J
5. H
6. B
7. E
8. A
9. G
10. D

REVIEW QUESTIONS—INSPECTION AND PALPATION (p. 191)

1. F
2. T
3. F
4. T
5. T
6. F
7. F
8. See Bates
9. See Bates

13

musculoskeletal system (spine and extremities)

TO THE STUDENT

Since the examination of the musculoskeletal system entails primarily inspection and palpation, these two will be considered together. Please note that examination of the extremities includes observation of the skin, hair and nails, vascular structure, and regional lymph glands. However, since these specific areas are covered in detail in other sections, they are omitted from this section, in which the primary focus is on the musculoskeletal system.

Recommended materials:

1 Alexander, Mary, and Brown, Marie. *Pediatric Physical Diagnosis For Nurses.* New York: McGraw-Hill Book Co., 1974

2 Bates, Barbara. *A Guide to Physical Examination.* Philadelphia: J. B. Lippincott Co., 1974

3 Blue Hill Educational Systems, Inc. *Pediatric Physical Examination—The Skeletal System* (Videotape: 25 minutes)

4 Blue Hill Educational Systems, Inc. *Physical Assessment Examinations—Musculoskeletal* (Videotape: 18 minutes)

5 J. B. Lippincott Co. *Visual Guide to Physical Examination—Musculoskeletal* (Film/videotape: 14:30 minutes)

6 three adults and three children (of various ages) who will allow you to examine their musculoskeletal systems.

BASIC KNOWLEDGE

Behavioral Objectives

The student will be able to:

1 answer in writing all *Review Questions*
2 define in writing the terms listed under *Definitions*
3 describe a systematic approach to performing this examination
4 label on a diagram, and on a living person, anatomical structures of the wrist and hand, shoulder, ankle and foot, hip, spine, elbow, and knee, according to Figures 13–1, 13–2, 13–3, 13–4, 13–5, 13–6, and 13–7
5 label on a diagram and demonstrate on a living person complete range of motion of all joints as illustrated in Figure 13–8.

Figure 13–1
Wrist and hand

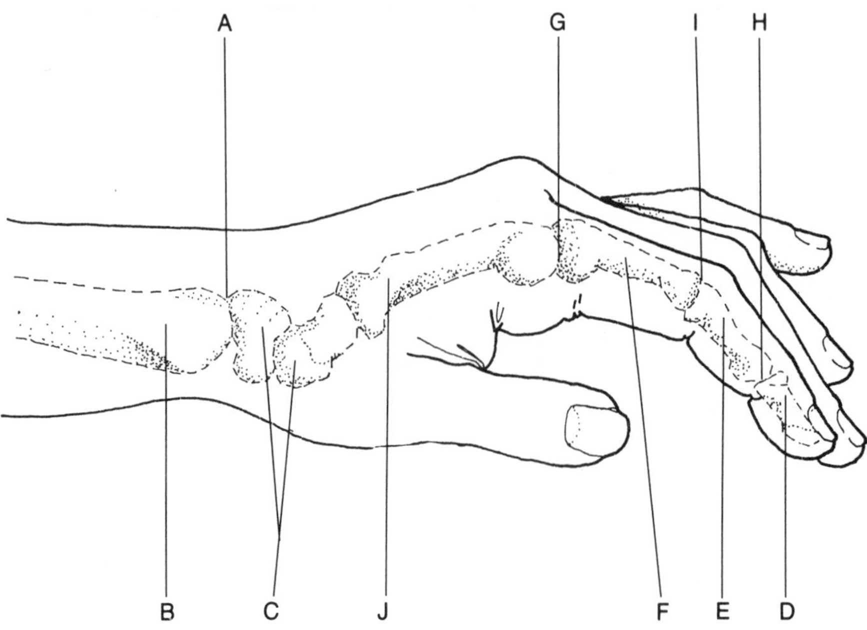

Label:

___ 1. distal phalanx
___ 2. middle phalanx
___ 3. proximal phalanx
___ 4. metacarpal
___ 5. carpals
___ 6. radiocarpal joint
___ 7. radius
___ 8. metacarpophalangeal joint
___ 9. proximal interphalangeal joint
___ 10. distal interphalangeal joint

Learning Activities

I Required

A *Read:* Alexander and Brown; Bates

B *Label:* Figures 13–1 through 13–7

C *Label:* Figure 13–8

II Optional

See listing of additional references and materials specific to musculoskeletal system in *Bibliography*.

Figure 13–2
Shoulder:

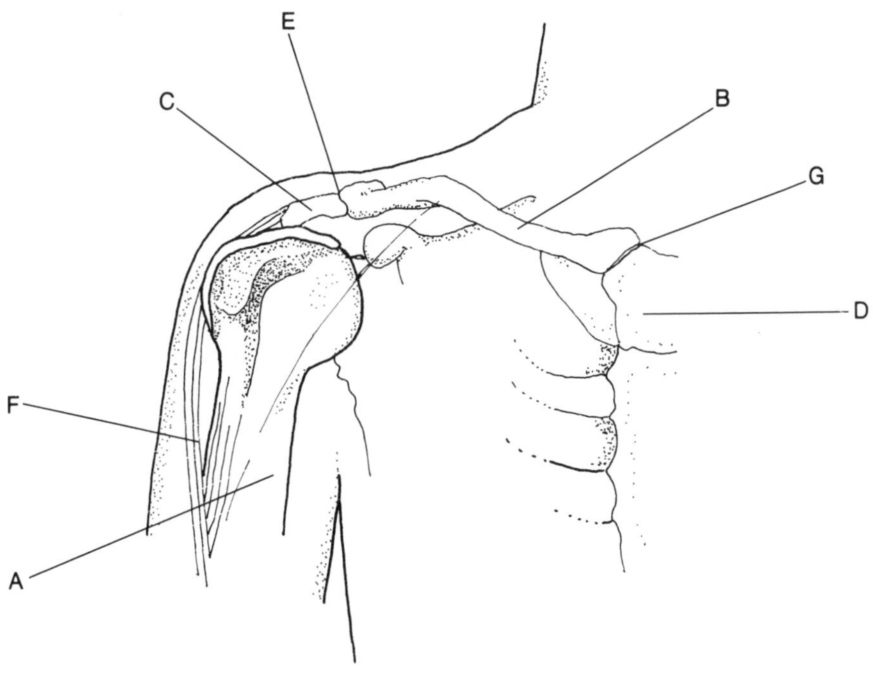

Label:

___ 1. manubrium of sternum

___ 2. sternoclavicular joint

___ 3. clavicle

___ 4. acromion

___ 5. humerus

___ 6. deltoid muscle

___ 7. acromioclavicular joint

Figure 13–3
Ankle and foot

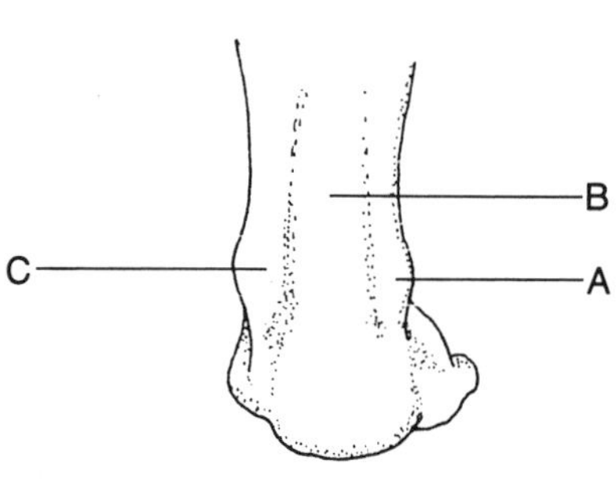

I.

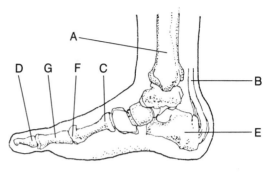

II.

Label:

____ 1. **medial malleolus**

____ 2. **Achilles tendon**

____ 3. **lateral malleolus**

Label:

____ 1. **Achilles tendon**

____ 2. **distal phalanx**

____ 3. **proximal phalanx**

____ 4. **tibia**

____ 5. **first metatarsal**

____ 6. **calcaneous**

____ 7. **metatarsophalangeal joint**

Figure 13–4
Right hip

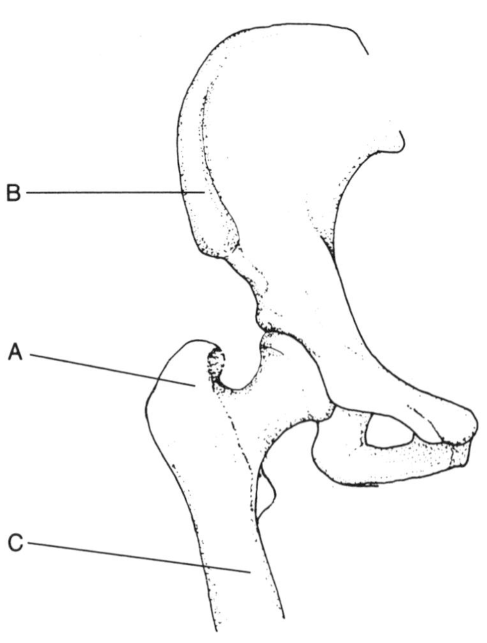

Label:

____ 1. **anterior-superior iliac spine**

____ 2. **greater trochanter**

____ 3. **femur**

Figure 13–5
The spine

Label:

___ 1. spinous process C_7

___ 2. spinous process T_1

___ 3. paravertebral muscles

___ 4. posterior-superior iliac spine

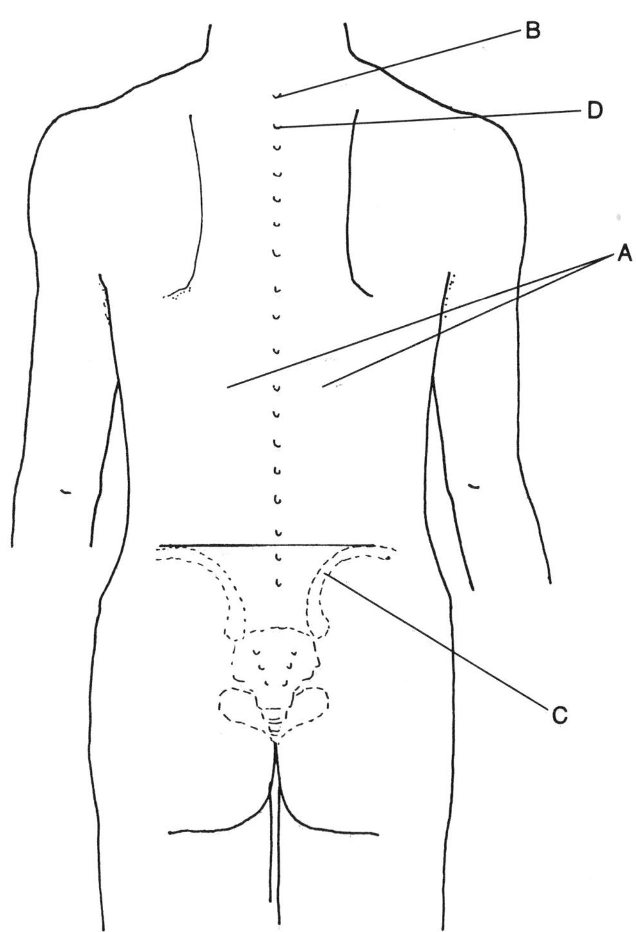

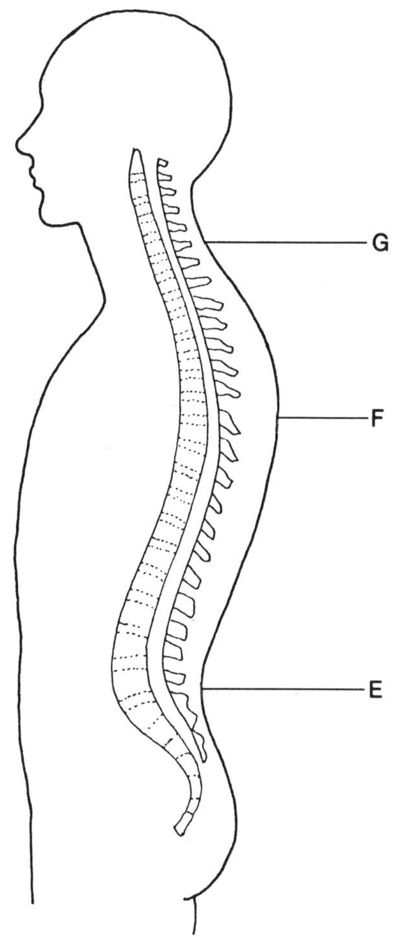

Label:

___ 5. cervical concavity

___ 6. thoracic convexity

___ 7. lumbar concavity

Figure 13–6
Left elbow

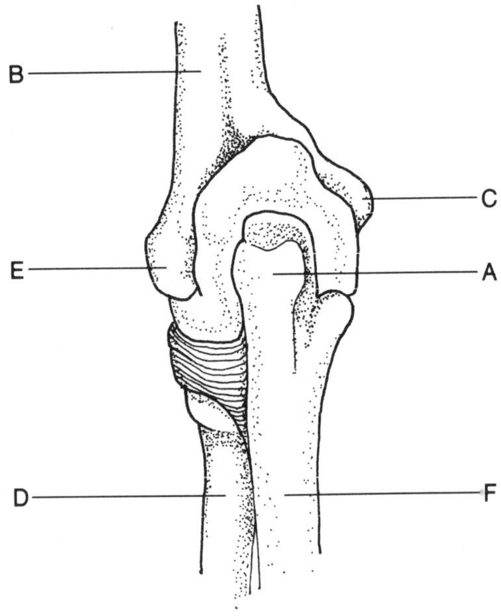

Label:

___ 1. humerus

___ 2. lateral epicondyle

___ 3. olecranon process

___ 4. medial epicondyle

___ 5. ulna

___ 6. radius

Figure 13–7
Left knee

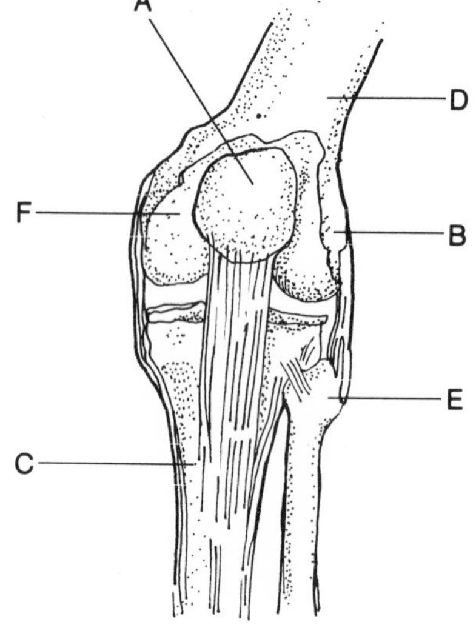

Label:

___ 1. femur

___ 2. lateral epicondyle

___ 3. patella

___ 4. medial epicondyle

___ 5. tibia

___ 6. fibula

Label the type of motion for each joint according to the arrows on the figures.

Figure 13–8
Range of motion

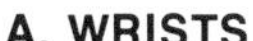

A. WRISTS

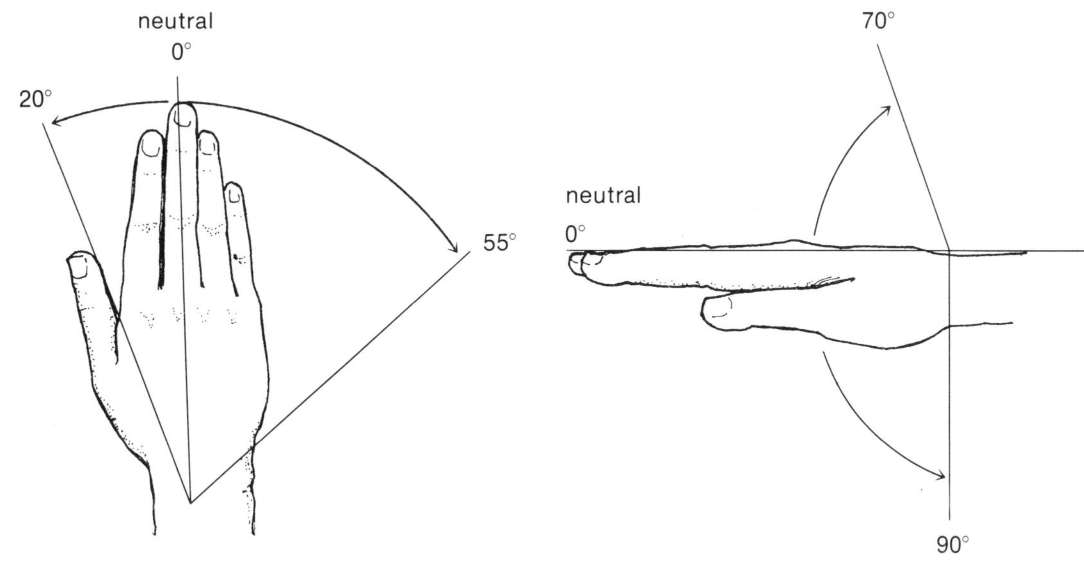

B. JOINTS OF FINGERS

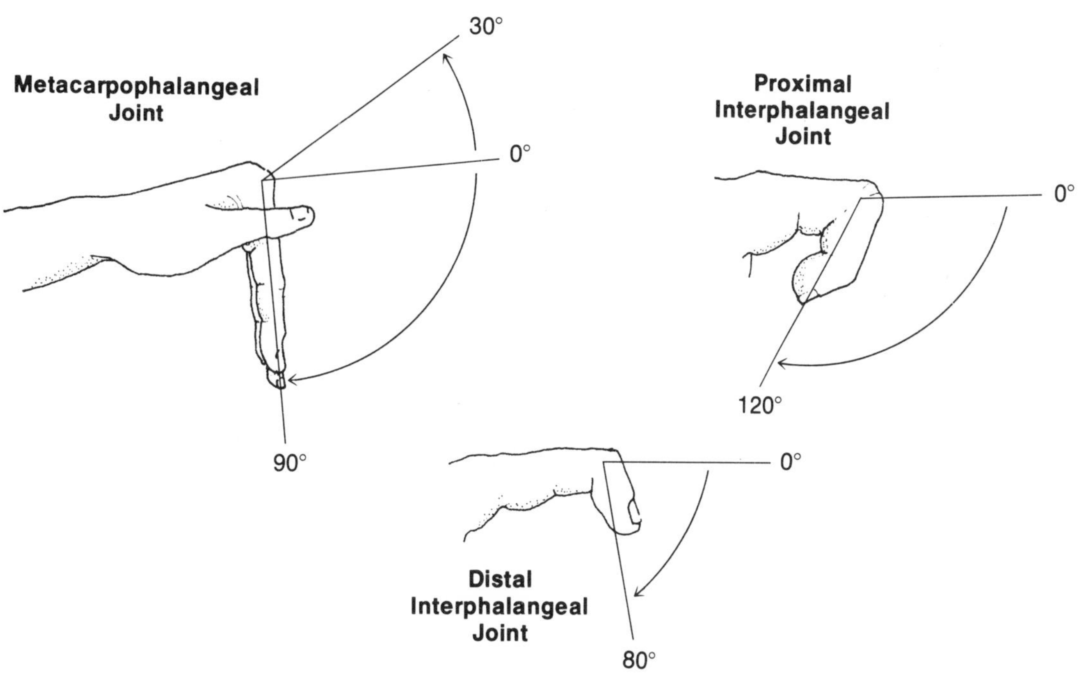

C. ELBOW

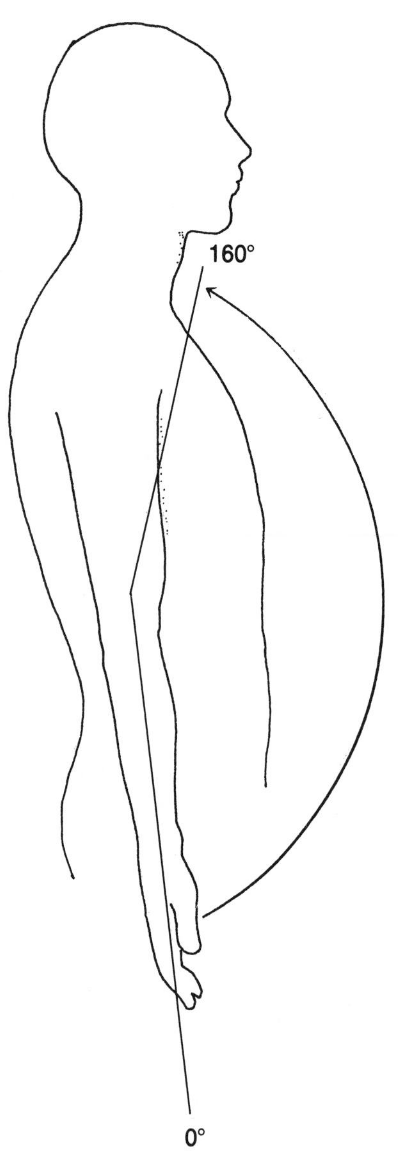

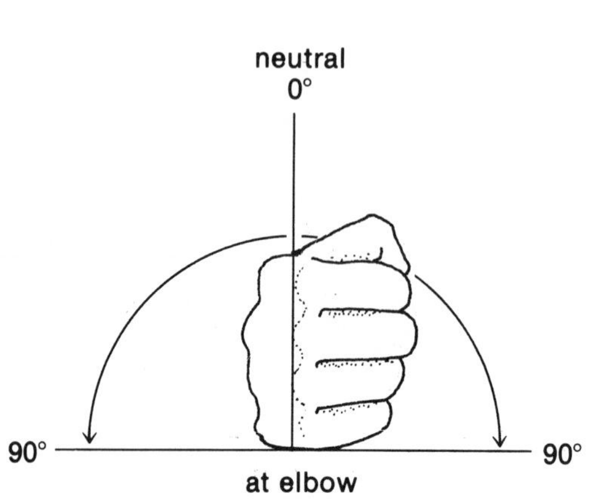

D. SHOULDER

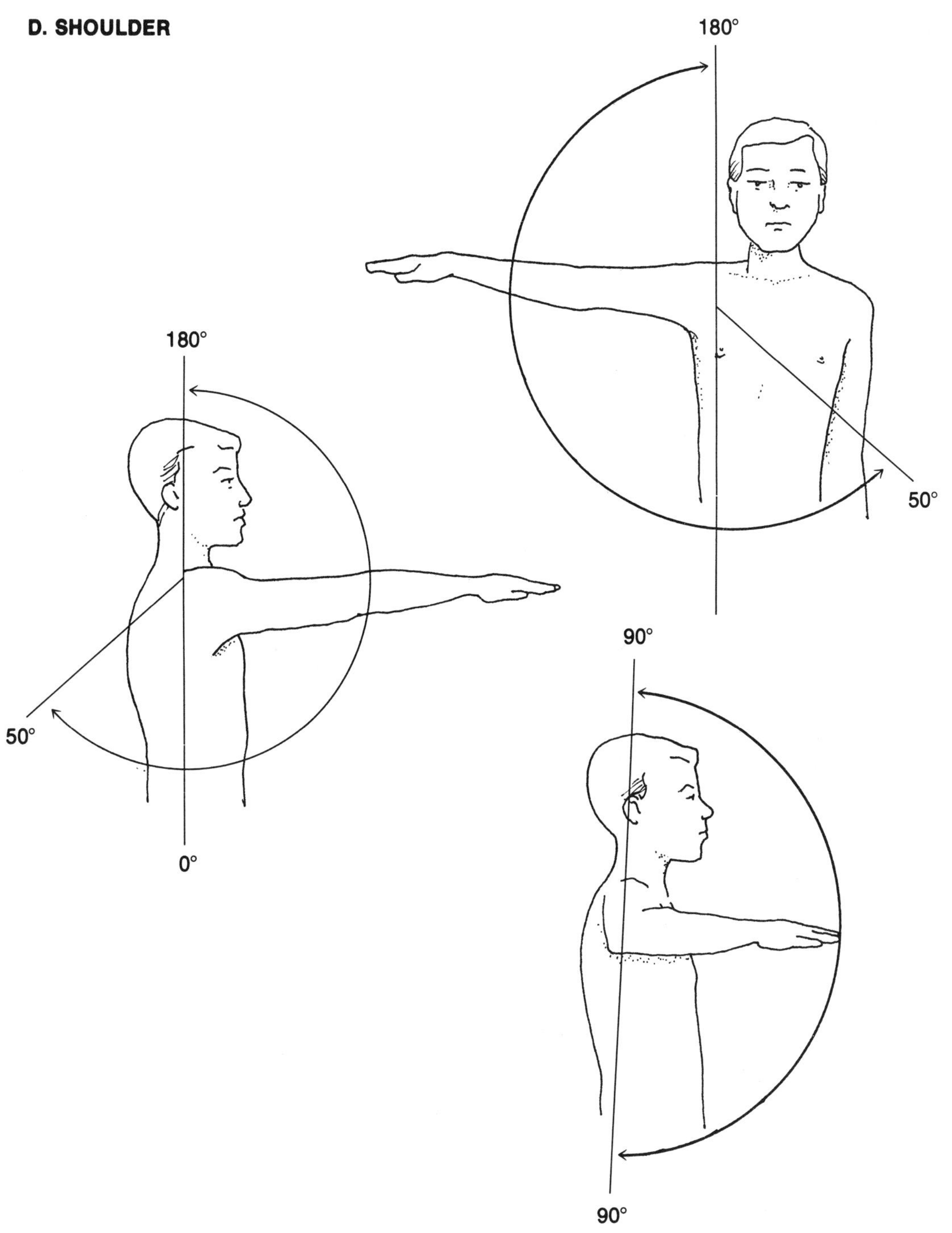

E. ANKLES AND FEET

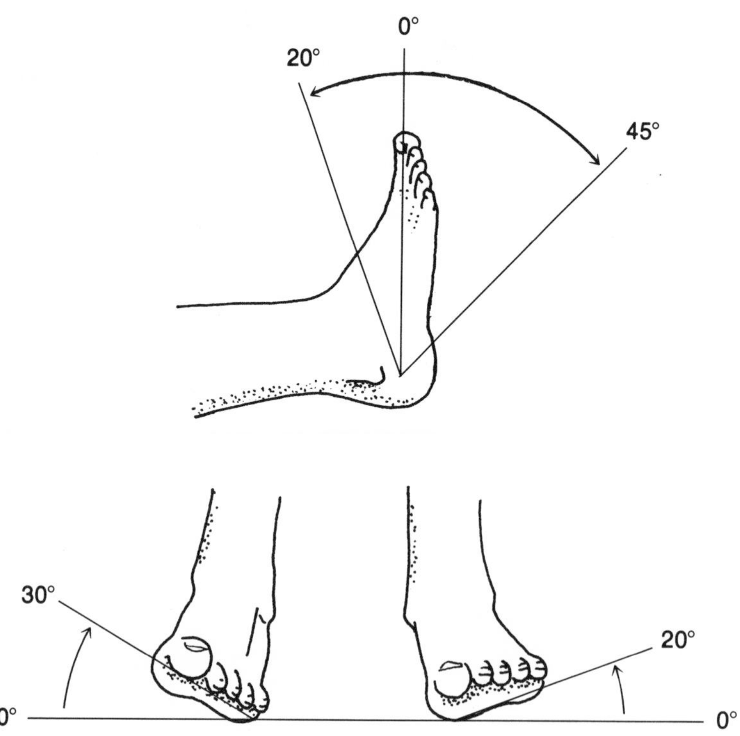

F. KNEE (right leg)

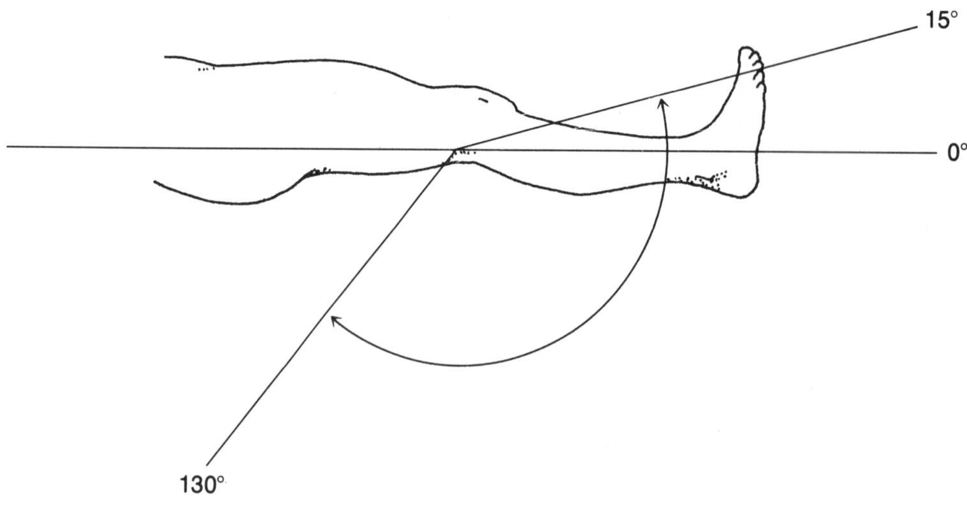

G. HIP

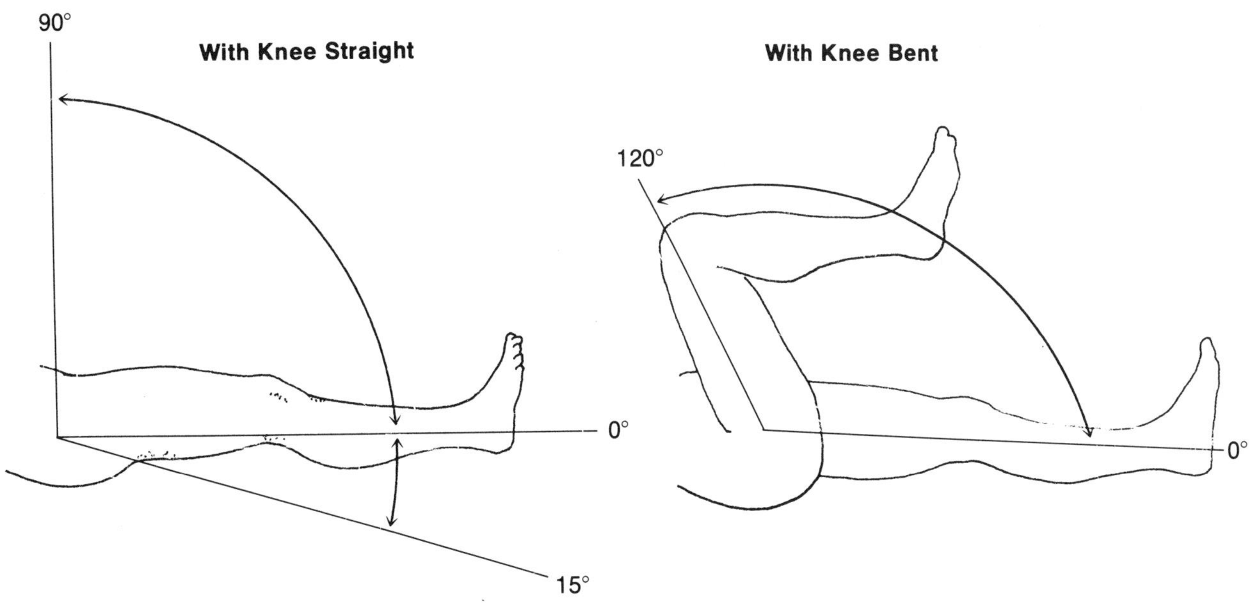

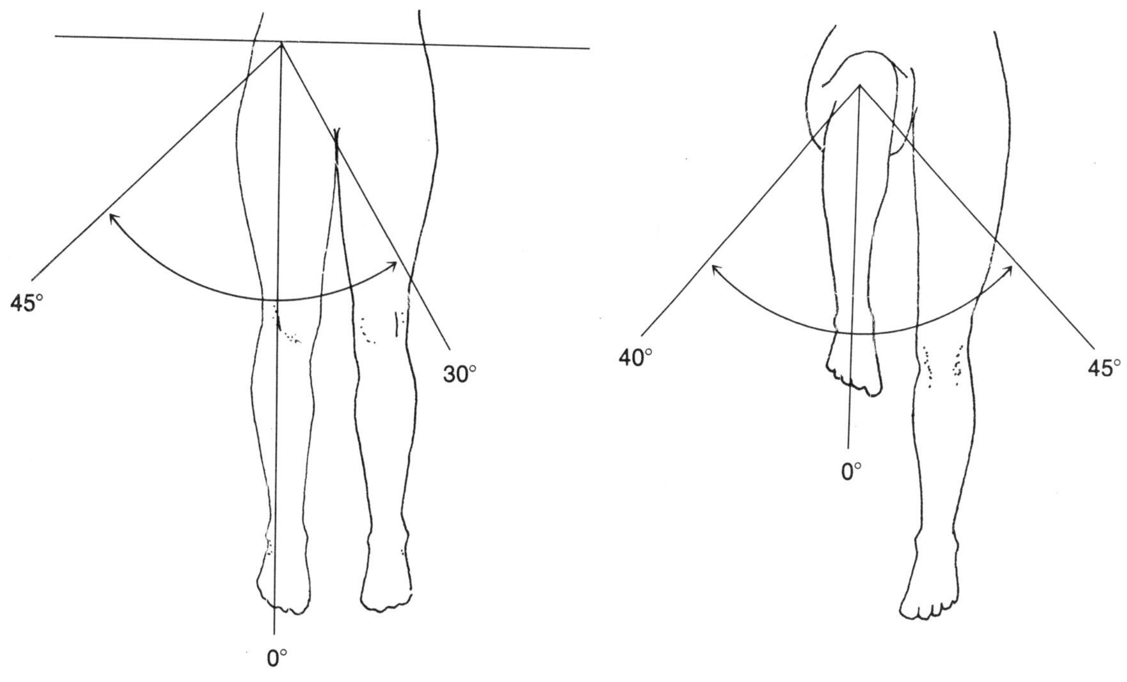

H. NECK

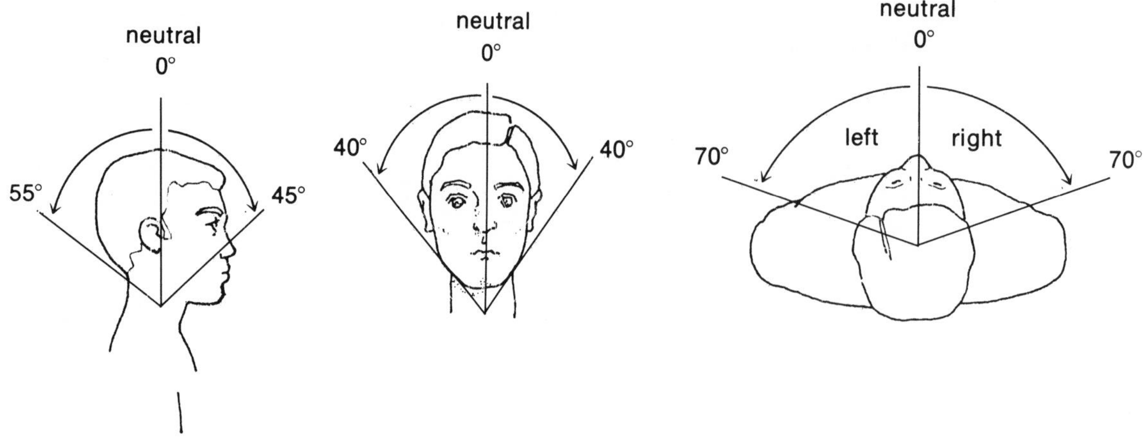

I. SPINE

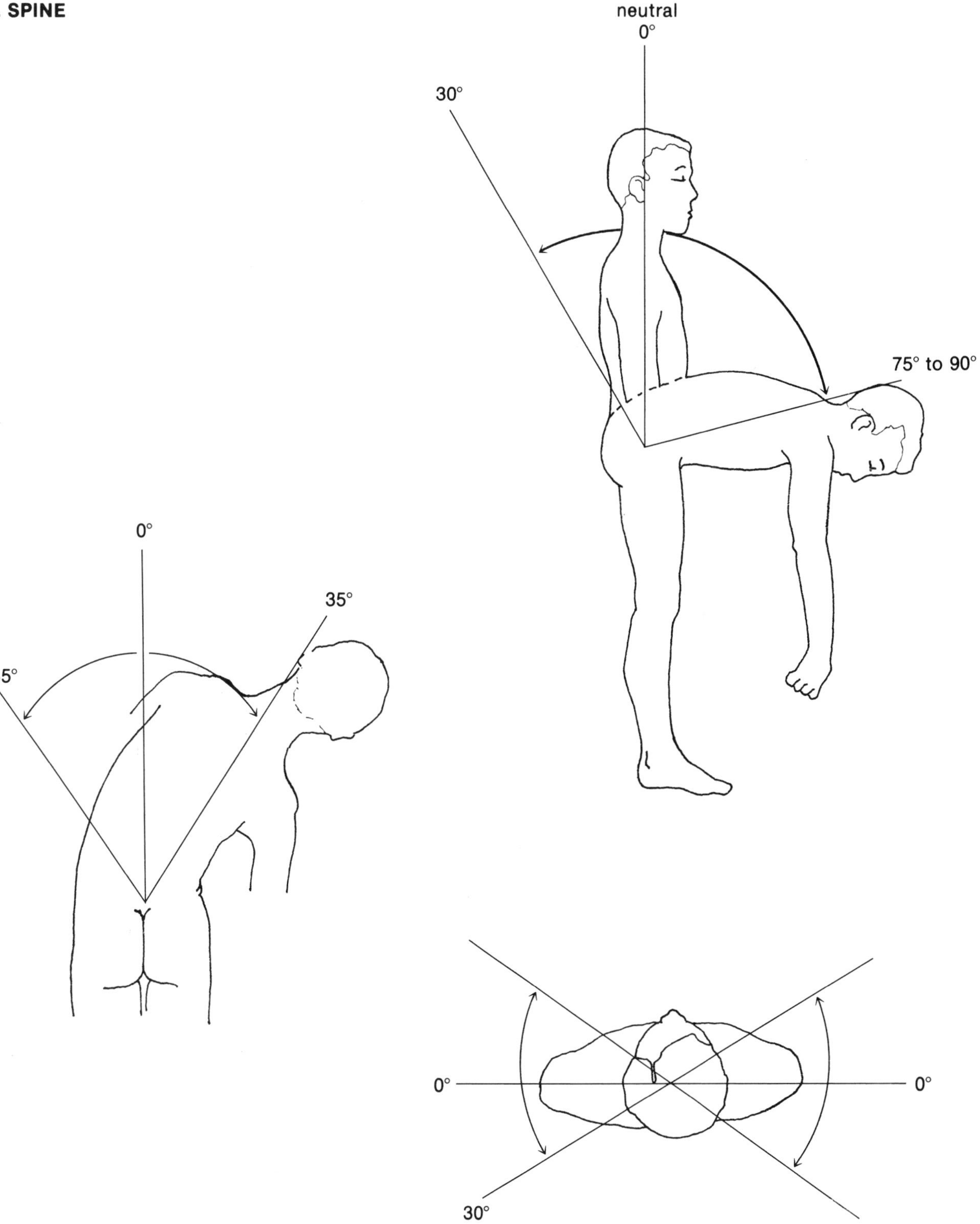

Definitions

Match the definitions in *Column I* with the correct words in *Column II.*

Column I

_____**1** turning the palmar side upward (referring to the hand); or with the face and abdomen upward (referring to the body)

_____**2** when referring to the body, the act of lying face downward; with respect to the arm, it is rotation of the forearm in such a way that the palm of the hand faces backward when the arm is in the anatomical position or downward when the arm is extended at a right angle to the body

_____**3** a turning outward

_____**4** a turning inward

_____**5** movement away from the midline

_____**6** movement of a limb toward the central axis of the body or beyond it

_____**7** movement of a part, as an extremity, in a circular direction

_____**8** the surface markings (sharply sculptured ridges) of the skin, especially of the palmar and plantar regions

_____**9** relating to the back; posterior

_____**10** relaxed, flabby, without tone

_____**11** any structure of angular shape, such as a flexed knee

_____**12** relating to the belly or abdomen; opposite of dorsal; anterior

_____**13** superextension; extension of a limb or part beyond the normal limit

_____**14** a movement that brings the parts of a limb into or toward a straight position

_____**15** range of motion of the patient's joints; (performed by another person—the patient does not actively move the joints)

_____**16** a closed sac lined with a membrane resembling synovium and containing fluid; often found in areas subject to friction; for example, over an exposed or prominent part or where a tendon passes over a bone

_____**17** turning of the foot or toes upward

_____**18** range of motion of a patient's joints when the patient actively moves the extremities, instead of having the extremities moved by another person

_____**19** the central cushion, of a gelatinous material, enclosed in several layers of fibrous tissue, lying within an intervertebral disk

_____**20** turning of the foot or toes downward

_____**21** an interarticular fibrocartilage of crescentic or discoid shape found in certain joints such as the knee

Column II

A genu
B passive range of motion
C nucleus pulposus
D supination
E meniscus
F extension
G pronation
H abduction
I plantar flexion
J eversion
K flaccid
L dorsiflexion
M inversion
N ventral
O bursa
P adduction
Q hyperextension
R active range of motion
S circumduction
T dermatoglyphics
U dorsal

Review Questions

TRUE—FALSE

Pediatric

_____**1** Only the thoracic and pelvic curves are present at birth.

Adult and Pediatric

_____**2** Pivot joints allow rotation only.
_____**3** The elbow is an example of a condyloid joint.
_____**4** The shoulder girdle includes the clavicle and scapula.
_____**5** The olecranon forms a major portion of the ankle.
_____**6** The carpal bones comprise the wrist.
_____**7** Each hand contains 14 phalanges.
_____**8** The femur does not become completely ossified before the fourteenth year of life.
_____**9** Growth in the length of the bone depends on growth of the periosteum.
_____**10** There are 33 connecting bones in the vertebral column.
_____**11** An example of a hinge joint is the movement of the humerus and ulna.
_____**12** The synovium of the elbow is normally palpable.
_____**13** The first two cervical vertebrae are known as the atlas and axis.
_____**14** The three to five bones of the coccyx become fused into one bone by age 15 years.
_____**15** The temporomandibular joint forms the articulation between mandible and skull.
_____**16** The radial nerve is located posteriorly between the olecranon and the medial epicondyle.
_____**17** The subacromial bursa lies between the deltoid muscle and the head of the humerus.
_____**18** The shin is the flat anterior surface of the fibula.

19 List the five groups of bones that form the vertebral column and the number of bones in each group.

INSPECTION AND PALPATION

Behavioral Objectives

The student will be able to:

1 answer in writing all *Review Questions*
2 identify each abnormality listed under *Definitions* by a picture or by a live example
3 state in writing how to assess one's ability to carry out the activities of daily living
4 state how to assess gait and deviations from a normal gait
5 assess the curvature of the spine and recognize abnormal curvatures
6 test for muscle strength in all extremities
7 examine each joint for thickened synovium, fluid, redness, heat, and tenderness
8 palpate for subcutaneous nodules and bone enlargements of each joint
9 examine the knee joint by looking for the bulge sign

10 test for tibial torsion and congenital dislocation of the hip
11 examine correctly for carpal tunnel syndrome of the wrist
12 check the knee for the audible click that is diagnostic of a torn meniscus
13 assess back pain for sciatica via straight leg raise
14 perform a total assessment of the musculoskeletal system on three adults and three children (of varying ages) and record findings appropriately, according to the check list provided.

Learning Activities

Required

A *Read:* Alexander and Brown; Bates

B *View:* Blue Hill Series videotapes *Pediatric Examination—The Skeletal System; Physical Assessment—Musculoskeletal*

C *Examine:* The musculoskeletal systems of three adults and three children (of various ages) and record your findings according to the check list provided.

CHECK LIST
Musculoskeletal System: Inspection and Palpation

Sex______________
Age______________

	Yes	No	Describe (*where appropriate*)
Ability to carry out ADL: able to walk, stand, sit up, rise from sitting position, lie down, pinch, climb, grasp, lean over (in child—jump and skip)			
able to comb hair, brush teeth, feed, wash, and dress self, carry out toilet hygiene, etc.			
Gait smooth, coordinated, rhythmic			
painful			
limp			
Spine all spinous processes palpable			
normal curvature			
abnormal curvature			
back pain/tenderness			
normal response to sciatic stretch test			

Length of extremities
- length same on both sides ______
- discrepancy between length of right and left sides (over 1 cm) ______

Joints (include all joints)
- pain or tenderness ______
- full range of motion ______
- abnormal mobility or unusual movements ______
- heat ______
- redness ______
- pain on motion ______
- crepitus ______
- discoloration ______
- effusion ______
- spasm ______
- swelling or deformity ______
- instability ______
- ankylosis ______
- thickened synovial membrane ______
- bony enlargement ______
- congenital defects ______

Muscle strength
- normal against gravity ______
- normal against resistance ______
- symmetrical for extremities ______

Condition of tissues surrounding joints
- muscle atrophy ______
- subcutaneous nodules ______
- skin changes ______
- swelling ______
- contractures ______

Definitions

Match the definitions in *Column I* with the correct words in *Column II.*

Part I

_____**1** a wasting of tissues, organs, or the entire body; e.g., the wasting of muscles due to disuse of a fractured limb

_____**2** the escape of fluid from the blood vessels or lymphatics into the tissues or a cavity

_____**3** lateral curvature of the spine

_____**4** an exaggerated anteroposterior curvature of the spine, generally lumbar, with the convexity pointing anteriorly

_____**5** stiffening or fixation of a joint

_____**6** an involuntary convulsive muscular contraction; cramp

_____**7** a curvature of the spine; humpback; hunchback; an abnormal curvature of the spine, with convexity backward due to caries and destruction of the bodies of the affected vertebrae

_____**8** an inflammatory swelling of the bursa over the metatarsophalangeal joint of the great toe

_____**9** an incomplete displacement or dislocation

_____**10** relaxed, flabby, without tone

A kyphosis
B effusion
C flaccid
D atrophy
E lordosis
F subluxation
G scoliosis
H spasm
I bunion
J ankylosis

Part II

_____1 a coarse, thick, square hand associated with acromegaly or myxedema

_____2 the sensation felt on placing the hand over the seat of the fracture when the broken ends of the bone are moved; also present when irregular surfaces are rubbing against one another, as in arthritis

_____3 nontender nodules in the subcutaneous tissues located around joints (elbows, knees) in individuals with rheumatoid arthritis

_____4 contraction of the palmar fascia, causing permanent flexion of one or more fingers

_____5 a circumscribed cystic swelling connected with a tendon sheath, due to shutting off of a hernial protrusion of the synovial lining of the sheath

_____6 paralysis of the extensors of the wrist and fingers due to lesion of the musculospinal nerve

_____7 pain and paresthesia (tingling, burning, and numbness) in the hand in the area of distribution of the median nerve; caused by compression of the median nerve by fibers of the flexor retinaculum

_____8 inflammation of one or more of the vertebrae

_____9 neuralgia of the sciatic nerve, felt in the back of the thigh

_____10 atrophy of the palm of the hand; often associated with carpal tunnel syndrome

_____11 permanent eversion of the foot, so that only the inner side of the sole rests on the ground; usually combined with a breaking down of the plantar arch

_____12 inversion of the foot, so that only the outer side of the sole touches the ground; there is usually more or less talipes equinus associated with it

A valgus deformity

B crepitation

C sciatica

D subcutaneous nodules

E spondylitis

F wristdrop

G spade hand

H thenar atrophy

I Dupuytren's contracture

J carpal tunnel syndrome

K varus deformity

L ganglion

Part III

_____1 permanent plantar flexion of the foot, so that only the ball rests on the ground; it is commonly combined with talipes varus

_____2 permanent dorsal flexion of the foot, so that the weight of the body rests on the heel only

_____3 joint enlargement with osteoarthritis due to trophic disturbances in patients with tabes dorsalis

_____4 a strain of the elbow with soreness of the forearm often caused by excess tennis playing; epicondylalgia externa

_____5 a fracture of the lower end of the radius with displacement of the hand backward and outward; an extension fracture

_____6 the presence of more than five digits on either hand or foot

_____7 webbing together of fingers or toes

_____8 abnormal enlargement of one or more fingers

_____9 a condition in which the movement of the finger is arrested for a moment in flexion or extension and then continues with a jerk

_____10 blood in a joint

_____11 when the patella (a large sesamoid bone in the combined tendons of the extensors of the leg that covers the anterior surface of the knee) is riding high on effusion of the knee

_____12 talipes equinus and talipes varus combined

_____13 valgus deformity

_____14 a deviation of the great toe toward the outer or lateral side of the foot

_____15 permanent flexion at the midphalangeal joint of one or more of the toes

A neuropathic joint
B floating patella
C syndactyly
D tennis elbow
E hemarthrosis
F Colles's fracture
G equinus deformity
H trigger finger
I polydactyly
J talipes calcaneous deformity
K hammer toe
L talipes equinovarus
M macrodactyly
N hallux valgus
O talipes valgus

Part IV

_____1 a twisting of the tibia usually resulting in an apparent pigeon toe walk
_____2 talipes valgus
_____3 an adduction of the feet often referred to as pigeon toe
_____4 deviation inwards of the forepart of the foot, usually associated with flat foot and accompanied by weakness and pain in the feet in the standing position
_____5 the uneven height of the 2 patellas when the person is lying on his/her back with knees totally flexed and feet flat on the table
_____6 a twisting of the upper leg bone often resulting in a knock-kneed appearance
_____7 a test for dislocation of the hip in the newborn in which the examiner flexes the infant's legs at the hips and bends the knees; in this position he proceeds to abduct the legs while keeping his fingers over the hip socket—a clicking sound or the palpable sensation of the femur slipping in and out of the socket indicates a possible dislocation
_____8 an orthopedic condition in which the metatarsal bones turn outward resembling Position I of the ballet dancer
_____9 a sharp, burning pain that follows a spinal nerve root distribution; associated with a diseased condition of the roots of spinal nerves
_____10 joint range of motion characterized by discontinuous, jerky movement; also characterized by sudden, brief halting or catching during movement
_____11 a deformity of the hand seen in patients with rheumatoid arthritis, characterized by hyperextension of the P.I.P. joint and hyperflexion of the D.I.P. joint
_____12 a cyst containing synovial fluid communicating with synovial fluid of the knee joint; also commonly known as Baker's cyst
_____13 extreme flexion of the toe; also referred to as hammer toe

A Ortolani's sign
B radicular pain
C claw toe
D pes varus
E swan-neck deformity
F femoral torsion
G cogwheel motion
H metatarsus varus
I popliteal cysts
J tibial torsion
K metatarsus valgus
L Allis's sign
M pes valgus

Review Questions

COMPLETION
(Fill in the blanks)

Pediatric

1 In the neonate, it is especially important to check for full range of motion of the shoulders in order to detect a common birth defect known as a __________.

2 If a three year old child complains of pain in his elbow and wrist and is unable to supinate his forearm, you might suspect __________ of the __________.

3 A low set thumb and a simian crease should cause the examiner to investigate the possibility of ______________________________.

4 If a small child spends a lot of time sitting in a T.V. squat, he may develop ______________________________.

5 A positive Allis's sign indicates possible __________________________ of the hip.

Adult

6 Bony enlargement of joints may indicate ______________________________.

Both

7 __________ and __________ are the primary methods of examination used in evaluating the musculoskeletal system.

8 Bilateral swelling, bogginess, heat, and tenderness of interphalangeal joints may indicate ______________________________.

9 A tender lateral epicondyle of the elbow may be indicative of __________.

10 __________ is present if the medial malleoli are more than one inch apart when the knees are touching.

11 Describe the method for measuring the length of the legs (i.e., state the landmarks used and the position of the patient).

12 How can you tell if the shortening of a lower extremity is *real* or *apparent?*

13 Describe one examination method for testing for tibial torsion.

14 Describe two methods for testing for congenital dislocation of the hip.

15 Describe one method for detecting fluid in the knee.

16 Describe a method for testing for carpal tunnel syndrome.

TRUE—FALSE

Pediatric

____**17** Apparent pes cavus may be normal in a young child.
____**18** Most children should be able to skip fairly well by age five or six.
____**19** Congenital dislocation of the hip is more common in girls than in boys.
____**20** Ortolani's sign is the least reliable test for a dislocated hip.
____**21** Pes valgus could be the cause of tibial torsion.
____**22** The child with metatarsus varus does not need to be referred.
____**23** A child with a protuberant abdomen could normally have a slight degree of lumbar lordosis.
____**24** If a child has functional scoliosis, the scoliosis will disappear when he bends forward to touch his toes.
____**25** The Trendelenburg test is positive when the pelvis rises on the side opposite to the weight-bearing limb.

Adult

____**26** In an adult, the thoracic spinal curve is normally convex.
____**27** In a right-handed adult, there may normally be better muscular development of the right arm than of the left.
____**28** Heberden's nodules are normal for the person over 55 years old.
____**29** Dupuytren's contracture prevents full extension of the fingers.

Both

____**30** It is important for the examiner to feel every area of the spine in order to detect the absence of spinous processes.
____**31** Normally, the spine has only one lateral curve.
____**32** When the patient bends to touch his toes, the lumbar spinous processes should separate.
____**33** The humerus and shoulder should normally move as a unit rather than separately.
____**34** Upon flexion of a normal hip, the lumbar spine should also move.
____**35** A ramrod or poker spine restricts movement of the spine in *all* directions.
____**36** The term "radiculitis" is synonymous with *sciatica.*
____**37** The patient may frequently confuse "hip pain" with low back pain.
____**38** A sustained position of flexion of the trunk is nearly always indicative of a back disorder.
____**39** The Lasègue test (sciatica test) is done by raising the leg with the knee flexed to determine irritation of either the nerve or the nerve root.

____40 If spondylitis is present, there will be decreased chest expansion during respiration.

____41 Back pain is normally produced by straight leg raising and is increased by dorsiflexion of the foot.

____42 Torticollis refers to a lateral deviation of the head and neck.

____43 A neurological examination of the upper extremities should always be performed on a patient with neck and radicular pain.

____44 Winging of the scapula can be detected by having the patient push against a wall with the flat of both hands while the examiner observes both scapulae.

____45 Cubitus valgus and cubitus varus usually result from healed supracondylar fractures of the humerus during childhood.

____46 Traumatic dislocation of the hip results in a deformity characterized by adduction, internal rotation, and flexion of the hip.

Self-Evaluation Key

FIGURE 13–1 (p. 194)

1. D
2. E
3. F
4. J
5. C
6. A
7. B
8. G
9. I
10. H

FIGURE 13–2 (p. 195)

1. D
2. G
3. B
4. C
5. A
6. F
7. E

FIGURE 13–3 (p. 196)

I Ankle

1. C
2. B
3. A

II Foot

1. B
2. D
3. G
4. A
5. C
6. E
7. F

FIGURE 13–4 (p. 196)

1. B
2. A
3. C

FIGURE 13–5 (p. 197)

1. B
2. D
3. A
4. C
5. G
6. F
7. E

FIGURE 13–6 (p. 198)

1. B
2. E
3. A
4. C
5. F
6. D

FIGURE 13–7 (p. 198)

1. D
2. B
3. A
4. F
5. C
6. E

FIGURE 13–8 (pp. 199–205; see pp. 219–225)

DEFINITIONS—BASIC KNOWLEDGE (p. 206)

1. D
2. G
3. J
4. M
5. H
6. P
7. S
8. T
9. U
10. K
11. A
12. N
13. Q
14. F
15. B
16. O
17. L
18. R
19. C
20. I
21. E

REVIEW QUESTIONS—BASIC KNOWLEDGE (p. 207)

1. T
2. T
3. F
4. T
5. F
6. T
7. T
8. T
9. F
10. T
11. T
12. F
13. T
14. F
15. T
16. F
17. T
18. F
19. cervical 7
    thoracic 12
    lumbar 5
    sacrum 5
    coccyx (1–4)

DEFINITIONS—INSPECTION AND PALPATION (pp. 210–213)

PART I

1. D
2. B
3. G
4. E
5. J
6. H
7. A
8. I
9. F
10. C

PART II

1. G
2. B
3. D
4. I
5. L
6. F
7. J
8. E
9. C
10. H
11. A
12. K

PART III

1. G
2. J
3. A
4. D
5. F
6. I
7. C
8. M
9. H
10. E
11. B
12. L
13. O
14. N
15. K

PART IV

1. J
2. M
3. D
4. H
5. L
6. F
7. A
8. K
9. B
10. G
11. E
12. I
13. C

REVIEW QUESTIONS—INSPECTION AND PALPATION (pp. 214–216)

1. fractured clavicle
2. subluxation; radius/ulna
3. Down's syndrome
4. tibial torsion
5. congenital dislocation
6. osteoarthritis
7. inspection; palpation
8. rheumatoid arthritis (synovitis)
9. tennis elbow
10. genu valgus
11. lower extremities: measure from iliac crest to malleoli
12. measure it
13. see assigned readings
14. see assigned readings
15. see assigned readings
16. see assigned readings
17. T
18. T
19. T
20. F
21. T
22. F
23. T
24. T
25. F
26. T
27. T
28. T
29. T
30. T
31. F
32. T
33. F
34. F
35. T
36. T
37. T
38. F
39. F
40. T
41. F
42. T
43. T
44. T
45. T
46. T

Figure 13–8

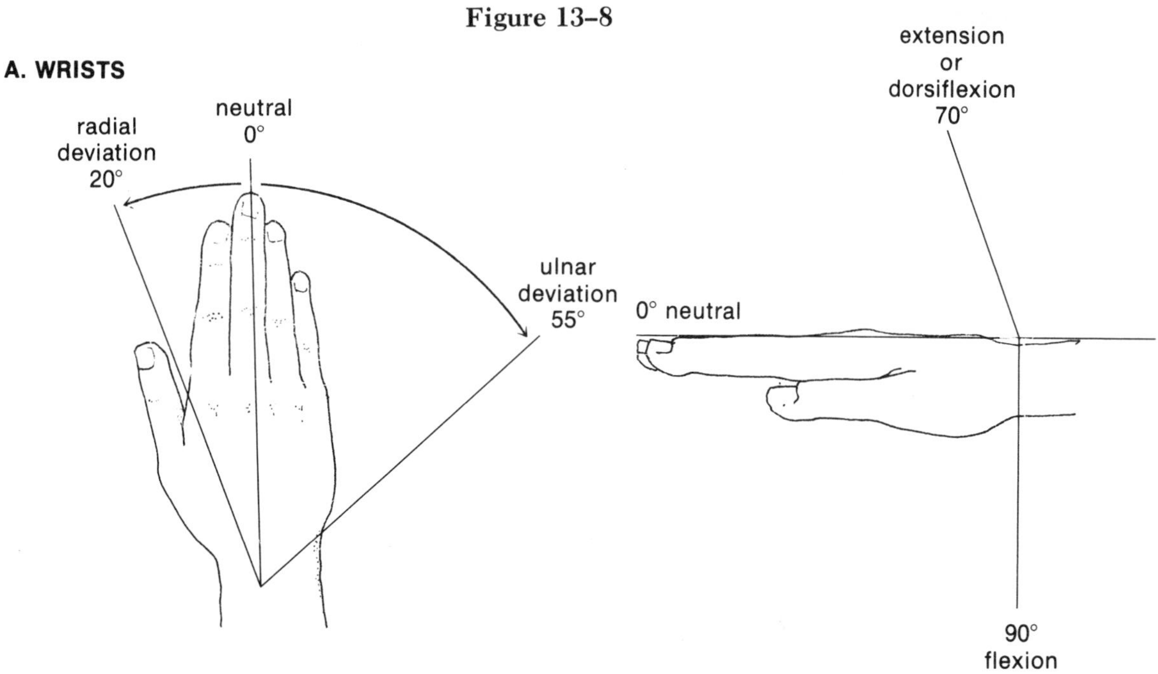
A. WRISTS
radial
deviation
20°
neutral
0°
ulnar
deviation
55°
extension
or
dorsiflexion
70°
0° neutral
90°
flexion

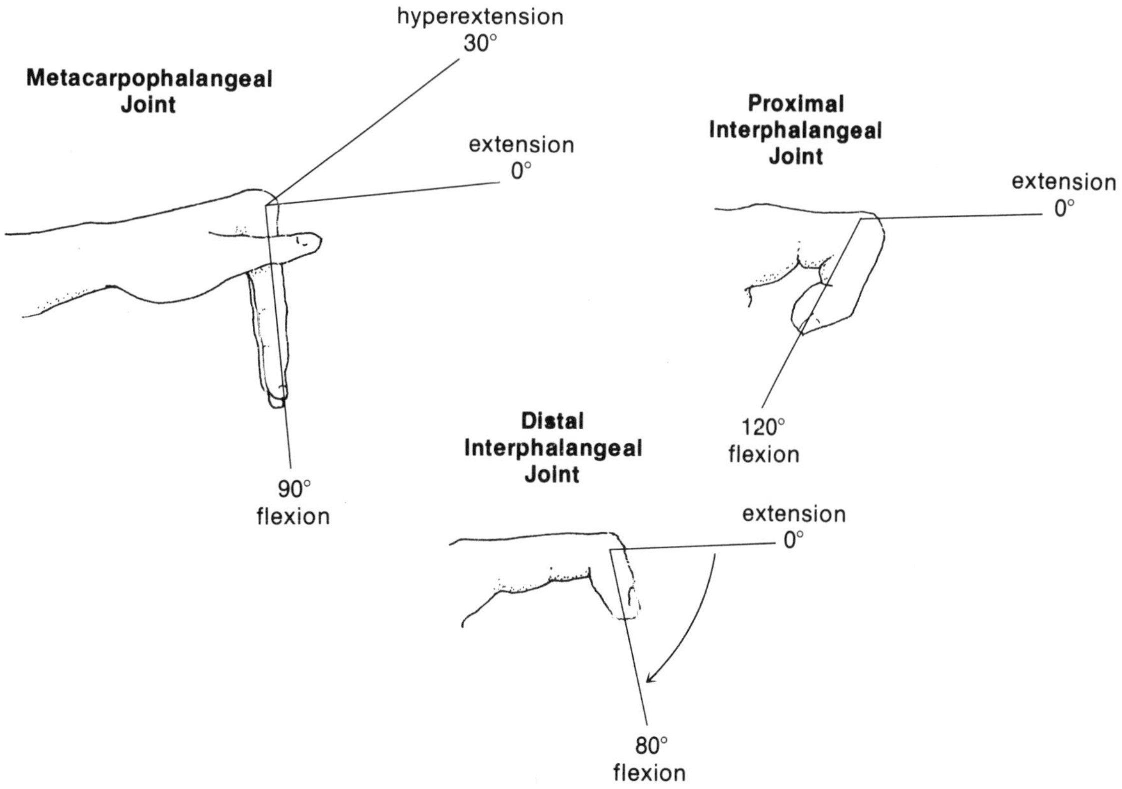
B. JOINTS OF FINGERS
Metacarpophalangeal
Joint
hyperextension
30°
extension
0°
90°
flexion
Proximal
Interphalangeal
Joint
extension
0°
120°
flexion
Distal
Interphalangeal
Joint
extension
0°
80°
flexion

C. ELBOW

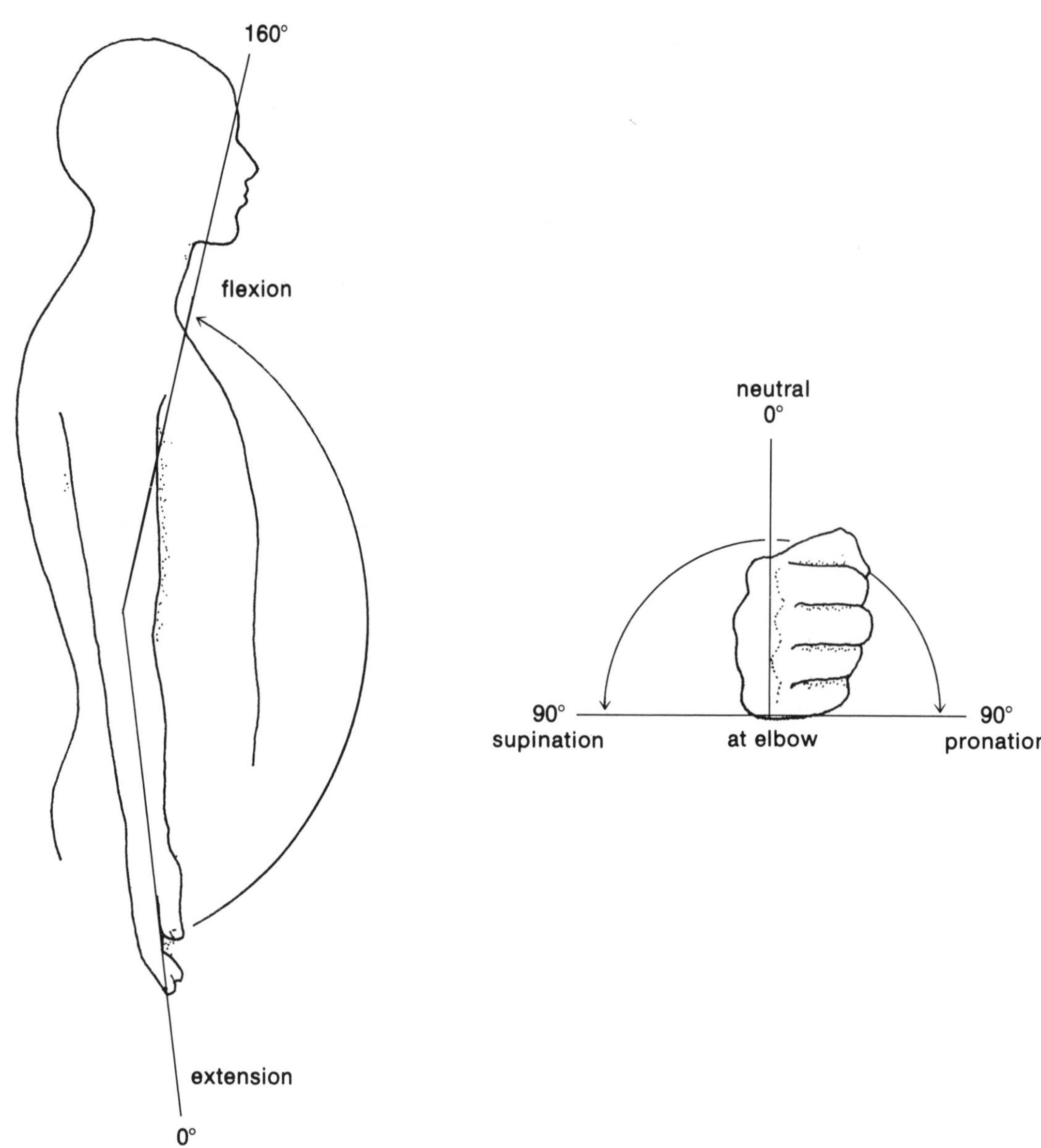
160°
flexion
extension
0°
neutral
0°
90°
supination
at elbow
90°
pronation

D. SHOULDER

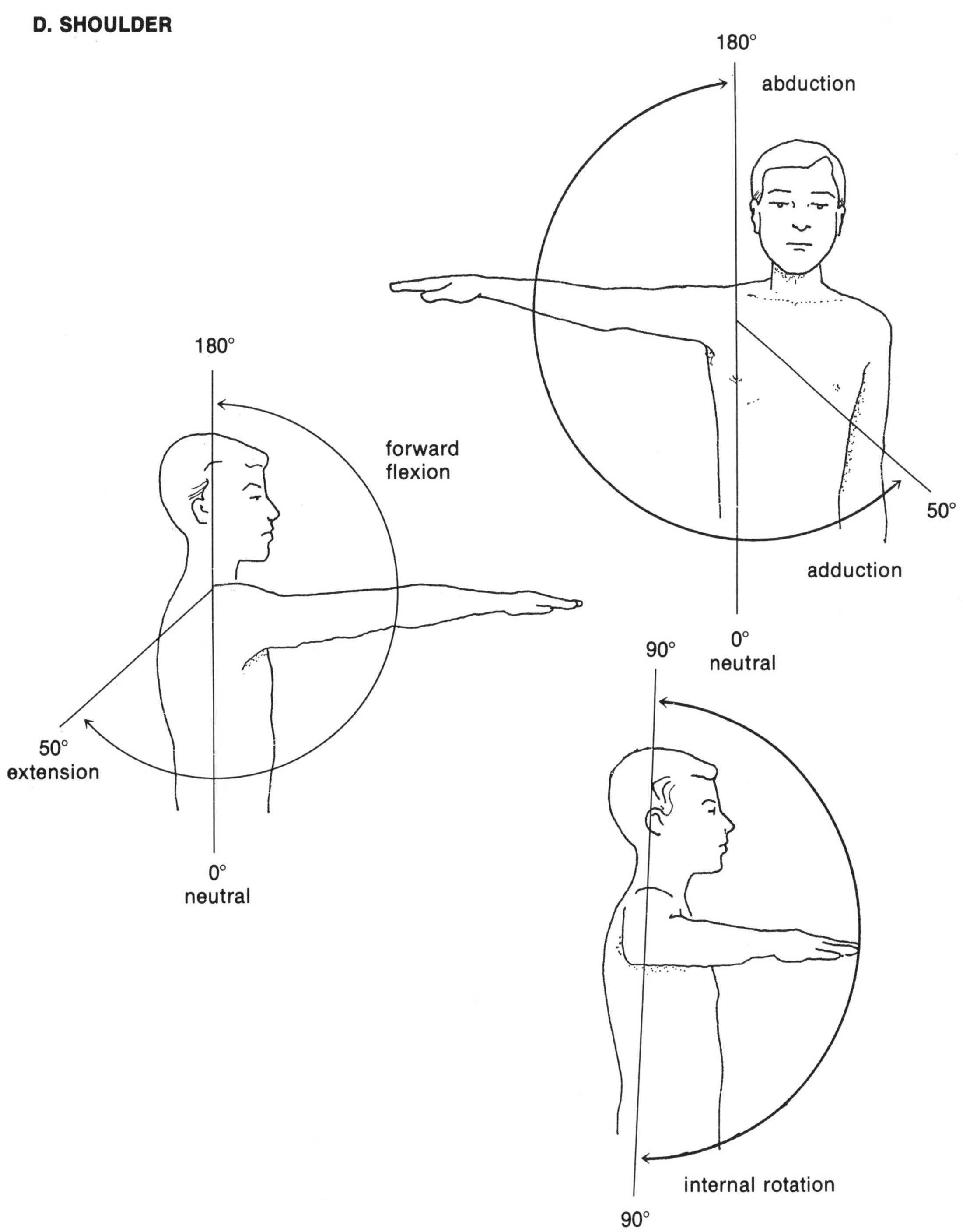
180°
abduction
50°
adduction
0°
neutral
180°
forward
flexion
50°
extension
0°
neutral
90°
internal rotation
90°

E. ANKLES AND FEET

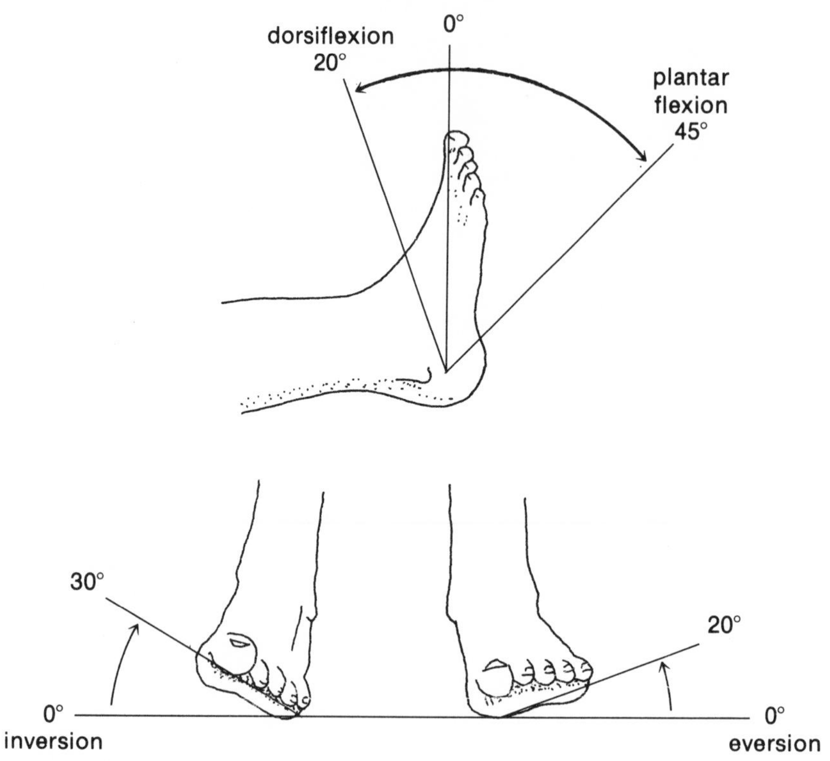

F. KNEE (right leg)

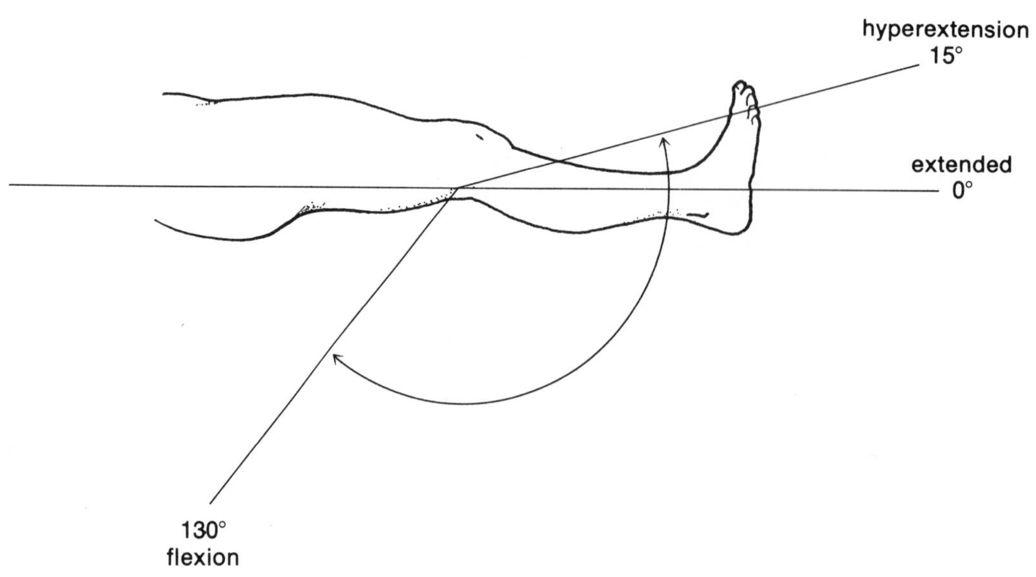

G. HIP

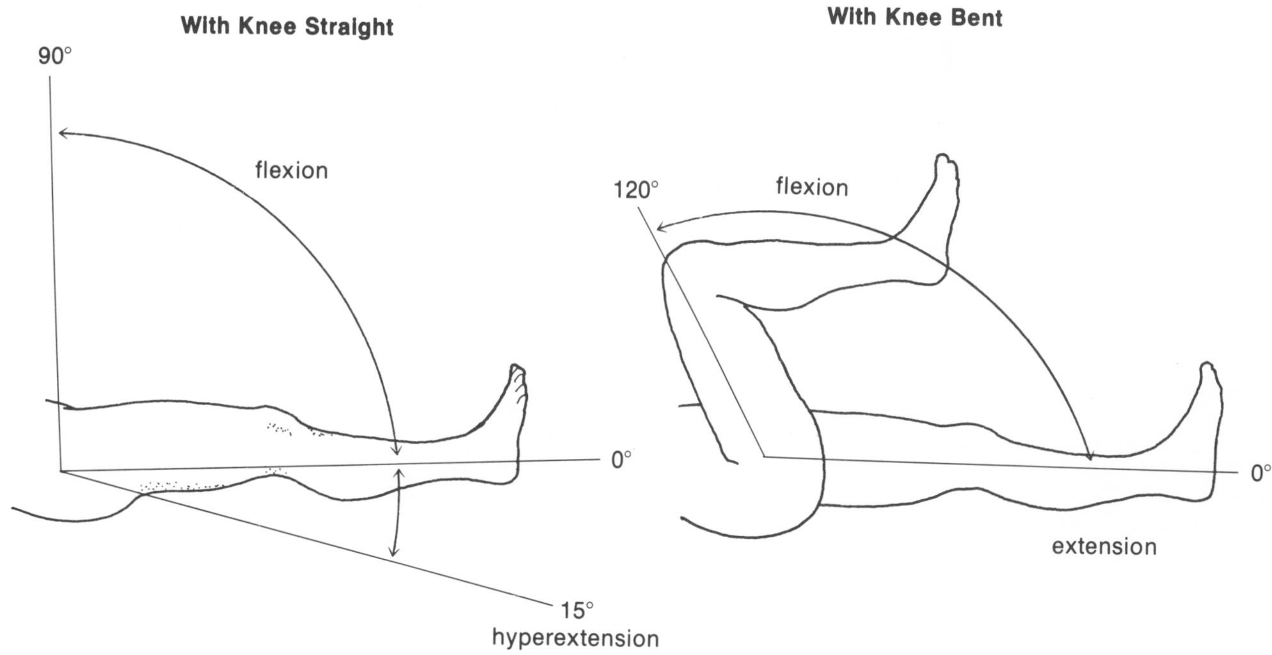
With Knee Straight
90°
flexion
0°
15°
hyperextension
With Knee Bent
120°
flexion
0°
extension

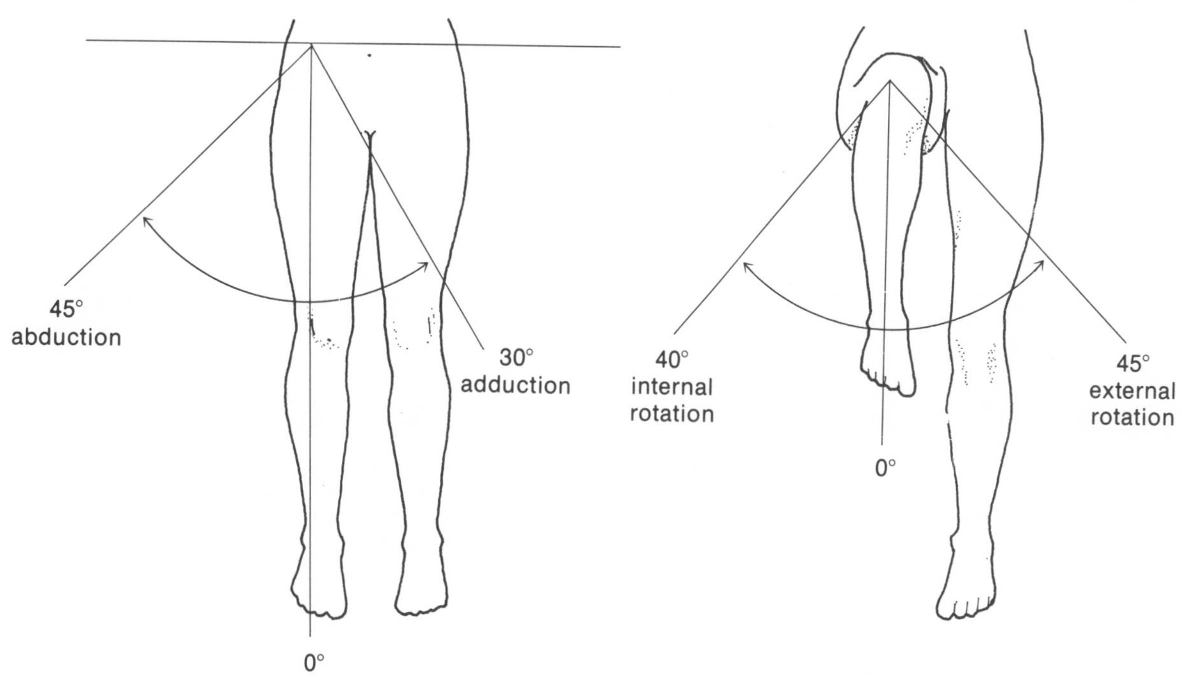
45°
abduction
30°
adduction
0°
40°
internal
rotation
45°
external
rotation
0°

H. NECK

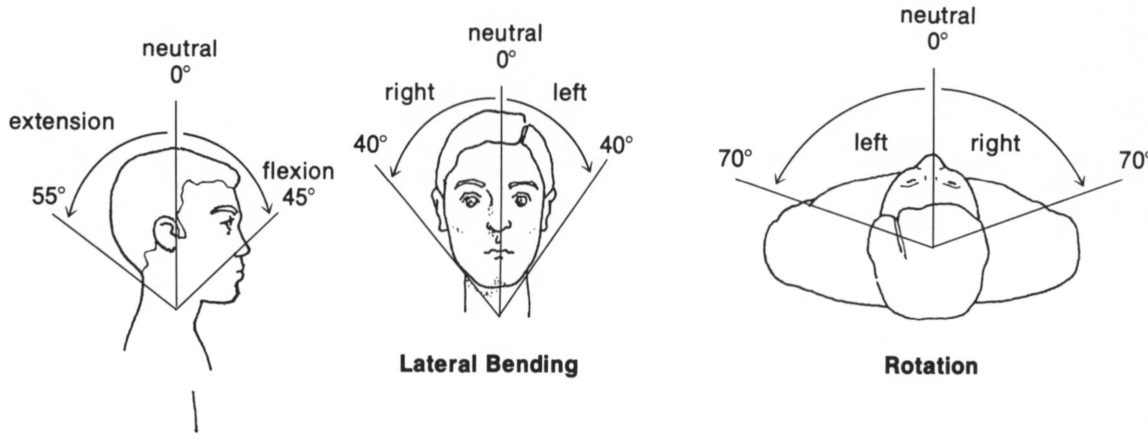

Lateral Bending

Rotation

I. SPINE

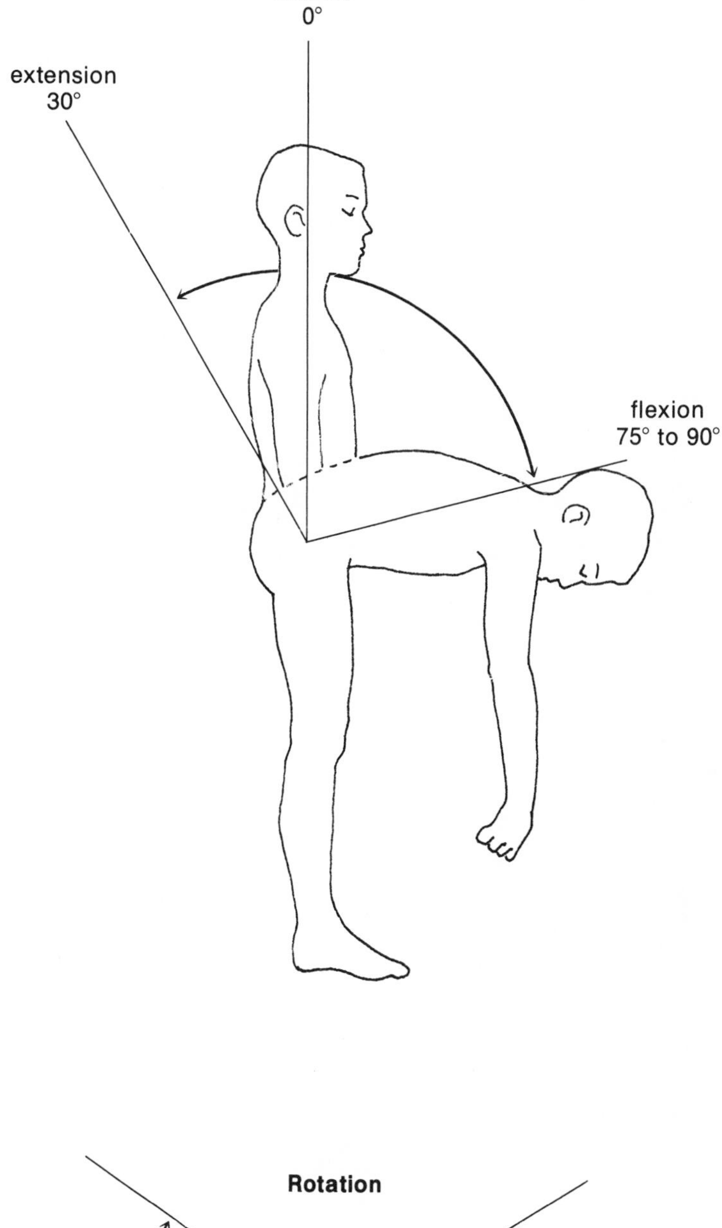

Lateral Bending

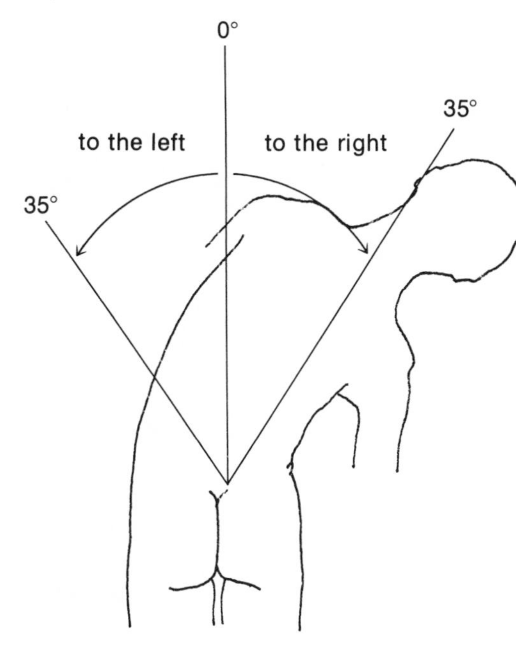

Rotation

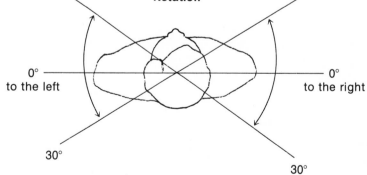

0°
to the left

0°
to the right

30°

30°

14

nervous system

TO THE STUDENT

This section is subdivided into six categories of the neurological examination, as outlined below:

1 Cerebral function (mental status and speech)
2 Cerebellar function
3 Motor system function
4 Reflex actions
5 Cranial nerve function
6 Sensory system function

Recommended materials:

1 Alexander, Mary, and Brown, Marie. *Pediatric Physical Diagnosis for Nurses.* New York: McGraw-Hill Book Co., 1974
2 Bates, Barbara. *A Guide to Physical Examination.* Philadelphia: J. B. Lippincott Co., 1974
3 "Patient Assessment: Neurological Examination, Part I." Programmed Instruction. *American Journal of Nursing* 75, no. 9 (September 1975): 1511–1536. Read also Part II, in *American Journal of Nursing* 75, no. 11 (November 1975): 2037–2062.
4 Blue Hill Educational Systems, Inc. *Pediatric Physical Examination—The Neuromuscular System—School-Age Child* and *The Neuromuscular System—Infant* (Videotapes: 50 minutes and 29 minutes)
5 Blue Hill Educational Systems, Inc. *Physical Assessment Examinations—Neurological* (Videotape: 55 minutes)
6 J. B. Lippincott Co. *Visual Guide to Physical Exam—Neurologic—Parts I & II* (Film/videotape: 35 minutes)
7 access to three adults and three children of varying ages who will allow you to examine their nervous systems.

CEREBRAL FUNCTION (MENTAL STATUS AND SPEECH)

Behavioral Objectives

The student will be able to:

1 answer in writing all *Review Questions*
2 define in writing the terms listed under *Definitions*
3 state in writing that evaluation of *general* cerebral function includes observations related to:
  a) general behavior and appearance
  b) level of consciousness
  c) intellectual or cognitive performance
  d) emotional status/mood
  e) thought processes and perceptions
  f) cortical sensory interpretations
  g) cortical motor integration
  h) language
4 state in writing that assessment of *specific* cerebral functions includes testing for:
  a) sound recognition
  b) auditory-verbal comprehension
  c) recognition of body parts and sidedness
  d) performance of skilled motor acts
  e) visual object recognition
  f) visual verbal comprehension
  g) motor speech
  h) automatic speech
  i) volitional speech
  j) writing
5 assess the cerebral function of three adults and three children of varying ages and record the findings appropriately, according to the check list provided
6 describe in writing the process for testing general and specific cerebral functions.

Learning Activities

I Required
  A *Read:*
    1 Alexander and Brown
    2 Bates
    3 *AJN* Programmed Instruction "Patient Assessment—Neurological Examination, Part II"
  B *View:* Blue Hill Series videotapes *Pediatric Examinations—The Neuromuscular System—School-Age Child* and *The Neuromuscular System—Infant;* and *Physical Assessment—Neurological*
  C *Examine and record findings* related to assessment of cerebral function of three adults and three children of varying ages
II Optional
  See listing of additional references and materials specific to neurological exam in *Bibliography*.

CHECK LIST

Nervous System: Cerebral Function

The following list should be filled in for each assessment of cerebral function required in the learning activities.

Sex____________
Age____________

	Describe Specific Behaviors and Responses	Indicate Tests Used	Evaluate Whether Response Is:		
			Normal	Abnormal	Questionable
I General cerebral function general behavior and appearance					
level of consciousness					
intellectual or cognitive performance					
emotional status/mood					
thought processes and perception					
cortical sensory interpretation					
cortical motor integration					
language					

	Describe Specific Behaviors and Responses	Indicate Tests Used	Evaluate Whether Response Is:		
			Normal	Abnormal	Questionable
II Specific cerebral function sound recognition					
auditory-verbal comprehension					
recognition of body parts; sidedness					
performance of skilled motor acts					
visual object recognition					
visual verbal comprehension					
volitional speech					
writing					
general impression					

Definitions

Match the definitions in *Column I* with the correct words in *Column II*.

Column I		Column II
_____1 an irresistible impulse to perform a certain act; usually the result of an obsession	A	phobia
_____2 a condition in which some one idea constantly fills the mind despite one's efforts to dislodge it	B	aphasia
_____3 any unreasonable or insane dread or fear	C	agnosia
_____4 a long-standing false belief or wrong judgment	D	compulsion
_____5 the mistaking of something for what it is not; when this is fixed and cannot be removed by evidence to the contrary it becomes a delusion	E	apraxia
_____6 a false perception having no relation to reality	F	delirium
_____7 a disorder of voluntary movement, consisting in a more or less complete incapacity to execute purposeful movements	G	obsession
_____8 a weakening or loss of the ability to use expressive or receptive language (e.g., reading, writing, speaking)	H	dysarthria
_____9 the appreciation of the form of an object by means of touch	I	hallucination
_____10 ability to recognize figures written on the skin	J	delusion
_____11 the sense perception of movement; the muscular sense	K	alexia
_____12 a specific type of aphasia limited to comprehension of visual language; "word blindness"	L	illusion
_____13 disturbance of articulation due to paralysis; incoordination or spasticity of the muscles used for speaking	M	stereognosis
_____14 a condition of extreme mental excitement marked by a rapid succession of confused and unconnected ideas, often with illusions and hallucinations	N	kinesthesia
_____15 lack of sensory ability to recognize objects	O	graphesthesia

Review Questions

TRUE—FALSE

_____1 A description of appropriateness of dress may be included in the assessment of cerebral function.

_____2 Unkempt appearance may indicate severe depression.

_____3 Dyslexia refers to reduced comprehension of the spoken language.

_____4 Orientation to time, place, and person is part of the assessment of the patient's intellectual or cognitive performance.

_____5 A question such as "Do you ever wish you were dead?" is a means of assessing mood or emotional status.

_____6 Normally, an adult should be able to repeat correctly at least ten numbers forward and eight backwards.

_____7 You could assume mental retardation any time a patient performs poorly on the digit span test and serial 7s.

_____8 Poor performance on abstract reasoning tests necessarily indicates thought disorders.

_____9 A question such as "What should you do if you are stopped for speeding?" is used to assess judgment.

____10 Having a patient close his eyes and identify an object placed in his hand is a test of his cortical motor integration.
____11 When the patient, with eyes closed, is asked to tell whether his finger is up or down, he is being tested for graphesthesia.
____12 Asking the patient the meaning of some common proverbs is a way of testing his ability to think abstractly.
____13 Compulsive behavior is frequently associated with obsessional thinking.
____14 Illusions are perceptual experiences, whereas hallucinations are distortions of actual perceptual experiences.
____15 Emotional lability is characterized by swings from crying to laughter and back to crying.
____16 In stupor, the patient is spontaneously unconscious but can be aroused sufficiently to respond to commands.
____17 Small word deletion in speech is known as telegraphic speech.

Pediatric

____18 Knowledge of normal development and knowledge of the child's previous behavior are the most important aids in evaluating his generalized cerebral function.
____19 A two- or three-year-old child's level of consciousness is primarily assessed via motor activity rather than verbal activity.
____20 A child of six years can generally repeat four digits forward.
____21 When a child is asked to take a piece of paper and seal it in an envelope, he is being evaluated for cortical motor integration.
____22 The quality of the infant's cry can be neurologically significant.
____23 Asking a child what he had for dinner last night is testing his recent memory.
____24 Children under five are developmentally too immature to be expected to compare two different weights.

CEREBELLAR FUNCTION

Behavioral Objectives

The student will be able to:

1 answer in writing all *Review Questions*
2 assess the cerebellar function of three adults and three children of varying ages and record the findings appropriately, according to the check list provided.

Learning Activities

Required

A *Read:*
  1 Alexander and Brown
  2 Bates
  3 *AJN* Programmed Instruction. "Patient Assessment—Neurological Examination, Part II"

B *View:* Blue Hill Series videotapes *Pediatric Examinations—The Neuromuscular System—School-Age Child* and *The Neuromuscular System—Infant;* and *Physical Assessment—Neurological*

C *Examine and record findings* related to assessment of the cerebellar function of three adults and three children of varying ages.

CHECK LIST

Cerebellar Function

The following list should be filled in for each assessment of cerebellar function required in the learning activities.

Sex____________
Age____________

Cerebellar Function	Describe Specific Response to Each Test Used	Evaluate Whether Response Is: Normal	Abnormal	Questionable
Upper extremities rapid rhythmic alternating movements				
point-to-point testing				
Lower extremities ability to stand on one foot				
gait and tandem walking				
Romberg test				
heel to shin test				

Review Questions

TRUE—FALSE

_____1 The cerebellum receives both sensory and motor input, coordinates muscular activity, and maintains equilibrium.

_____2 Motor skills such as handling a pencil and buttoning can indicate cerebellar function.

_____3 Consistent past-pointing in touching the finger to the nose and to the examiner's finger is probably indicative of a cerebellar problem.

_____4 The finger-to-thumb test is one way to test for rapid rhythmic alternating movements.

_____5 Awkwardness in running each heel down the opposite shin may indicate cerebellar disease.

_____6 Lesions in the cerebellum may cause staggering and falling.

_____7 Heel-to-toe walking in a straight line is usually done poorly in cerebellar disease.

_____8 The Romberg test involves asking the patient to stand with feet together and arms outstretched, with eyes open, then closed.

Pediatric

_____9 A child under four years of age with normal cerebellar function should draw a + sign without changing hands to cross the midline.

_____10 A four-year-old child should normally be able to stand on one foot for about five seconds.

_____11 Evaluation of cerebellar function in the two-month-old child includes assessment of coordination in reaching and grasping.

MOTOR SYSTEM FUNCTION

Behavioral Objectives

The student will be able to:

1 answer in writing all *Review Questions*

2 state in writing that evaluation of the motor system includes assessment of muscle size, muscle strength, muscle tone, and any abnormal muscle movements

3 assess the motor system function of three adults and three children of varying ages, and record the findings appropriately, according to the check list provided.

Learning Activities

Required

A *Read:*

1 Alexander and Brown

2 Bates

3 *AJN* Programmed Instruction. "Patient Assessment—Neurological Examination, Part II"

B *View:* Blue Hill Series videotapes *Pediatric Examination—The Neuromuscular System—School-Age Child* and *The Neuromuscular System—Infant;* and *Physical Assessment—Neurological*

C *Examine and record findings* related to assessment of motor system function of three adults and three children of varying ages.

CHECK LIST

Motor System Function

The following list should be filled in for each assessment of motor system function required in the learning activities.

Sex______________

Age______________

Muscle Group		Muscle Size	Muscle Tone	Muscle Strength	Abnormal Movement	Evaluate Whether Response Is: Normal	Abnormal	Questionable
neck								
upper arm	R							
	L							
lower arm	R							
	L							
wrist	R							
	L							
fingers	R							
	L							
thigh	R							
	L							
calf	R							
	L							
ankle	R							
	L							
toes	R							
	L							

Definitions

Match the definitions in *Column I* with the correct words in *Column II.*

____1 involuntary contraction or twitching of groups of muscle fibers; a coarser form of muscular contraction than fibrillation

____2 facial irritability in tetany; unilateral spasm can be excited by a slight tap over the facial nerve

____3 in latent tetany, typical attitude of the hand that is assumed when the upper arm is compressed, as by a tourniquet or blood pressure cuff

____4 a state of abnormal (either hypo- or hyper-) tonicity in any of the tissues

____5 contraction of the muscles that maintain a person in the standing position, following transection of the brain

____6 trembling or shaking

____7 flapping tremor of the hands; a characteristic abnormality of movement that occurs in advanced stages of liver disease, particularly in association with hepatic coma; it may also occur in diffuse cerebral disturbances of metabolism

____8 a condition in which there is a constant succession of slow, writhing, involuntary movements of flexion, extension, pronation, and supination of the fingers and hands, and sometimes of the toes and feet

A tremors
B athetosis
C fasciculations
D decerebrate rigidity
E Trousseau's sign
F asterixis
G Chvostek's sign
H dystonia

Review Questions

TRUE—FALSE

Pediatric

_____**1** Either hypertrophy or atrophy of the muscles might be associated with muscular dystrophy in the child.

Adult

_____**2** Parkinson's tremor increases with voluntary movement.

Both

_____**3** If there is any question as to asymmetry of muscle size of limbs, measurements should be taken.

_____**4** Flexion of the thigh at the hip is tested with the patient in a prone position.

_____**5** Muscle strength depends to some degree on age.

_____**6** Normal patients can contract their muscles promptly and maximally on command.

_____**7** The examiner should test homologous muscles simultaneously.

_____**8** The best way to test muscle strength is to have the patient place a limb in the described position and resist the examiner's attempt to displace it.

_____**9** The strength of the neck flexor is assessed by the resistance encountered when the examiner's hand is placed against the back of the patient's head.

_____**10** The strength of the finger flexors is estimated by the effort necessary to straighten the flexed fingers of the patient.

_____**11** Strength of adduction of the arms is tested by having the patient resist abduction.

_____**12** Strength of the abdominal muscles and flexors is evaluated as the patient attempts to sit up from the supine position.

_____**13** Plantar flexion is tested by having the patient push his foot down against the examiner's hand.

_____**14** Patients with impairment of proprioception show increased swaying and unsteadiness on their feet when their eyes are closed.

ANSWER CHOICE

(Choose the correct answer in parentheses)

Pediatric

15 For the first two months, an infant's muscle tone is expected to be primarily of the (**a** *flexor;* **b** *extensor*) type.

16 As a child's muscles enter the stage of (**a** *extension;* **b** *flexion*), spasticity may begin to appear in the case of cerebral palsy.

17 When a child with beginning signs of cerebral palsy has his head pushed forward, he will frequently (**a** *drop his head;* **b** *resist the pressure*).

Adult and Pediatric

18 A resting tremor is (**a** *diminished;* **b** *accentuated*) by voluntary movement.

REFLEX ACTIONS

Behavioral Objectives

The student will be able to:

1 answer in writing all *Review Questions*
2 state in writing how to elicit each of the deep tendon reflexes and the superficial reflexes, as listed on the check list
3 state in writing the criteria for grading reflexes according to the 0 to 4+ scale
4 state which reflexes are normal or abnormal according to age (see check list)
5 describe in writing the reflex arc
6 assess the reflex action of three adults and three children of varying ages and record the findings appropriately, according to the check list provided.

Learning Activities

Required

A *Read:*
  1 Alexander and Brown
  2 Bates
  3 *AJN* Programmed Instruction. "Patient Assessment—Neurological Examination, Part II"

B *View:* Blue Hill Series videotapes *Pediatric Examinations—The Neuromuscular System—School-Age Child* and *The Neuromuscular System—Infant;* and *Physical Assessment—Neurological*

C *Examine and record findings* related to assessment of the reflex actions of three adults and three children of varying ages.

CHECK LIST

Reflex Actions

The following list should be filled in for each assessment of reflex action required in the learning activities.

Sex____________
Age____________

Reflex Actions	Rate According to the 0 to 4+ Scale Describe (*where appropriate*)	Evaluate Whether Response Is:		
		Normal	Abnormal	Questionable
Deep reflexes (adult and child) biceps R.				
L.				
brachioradialis R.				
L.				
triceps R.				
L.				
patellar (knee) R.				
L.				
Achilles R.				
L.				
Superficial reflexes upper abdominal				
lower abdominal				
plantar R.				
L.				
Abnormal reflexes Babinski R.				
L.				

Reflex Actions	Rate According to the 0 to 4+ Scale Describe (*where appropriate*)	Evaluate Whether Response Is:		
		Normal	Abnormal	Questionable
Other reflexes (related to the infant only)				
acoustic blink reflex				
tonic neck reflex				
recoil of the arm				
ankle clonus				
palmar grasp reflex				
crossed extensor reflex				
withdrawal reflex				
rooting reflex				
sucking reflex				
Moro reflex				
Galant's reflex				
placing reflex				
stepping reflex				
Landau reflex				
parachute reflex				
Additional superficial reflexes (for children and/or the adult)				
abdominal				
RUQ				
RLQ				
LUQ				
LLQ				
cremasteric				
R.				
L.				
plantar group				
Other abnormal reflexes (for either child or adult)				
Chaddock				
R.				
L.				
Oppenheim				
R.				
L.				
Gordon				
R.				
L.				
Chvostek's reflex				

Review Questions

Word Choice

(Choose the correct answer in the parentheses)

Adult and Pediatric

1 The patellar reflex should show a normal response of knee (**a** *extension;* **b** *flexion*).

2 A deep tendon reflex (**a** *is;* **b** *is not*) dependent upon an intact motor nerve fiber.

3 Reflex activity (**a** *is;* **b** *is not*) dependent upon cerebral cortex function.

4 A grade of 4+ on reflex activity could be described as a/an (**a** *normal;* **b** *abnormal*) response.

5 In eliciting the deep tendon reflexes it is important to position the limbs so that the muscle is mildly (**a** *stretched;* **b** *contracted*).

6 Extension of the elbow is the normal response of the (**a** *triceps;* **b** *biceps*) reflex.

7 (**a** *plantar;* **b** *dorsi-*) flexion of the foot is the normal response to the Achilles reflex.

8 If present, ankle (**a** *clonus;* **b** *tonus*) may be elicited by suddenly and briskly dorsiflexing the foot and applying sustained, moderate pressure.

9 The normal response in terms of the upper abdominal reflex is that the umbilicus moves (**a** *down,* **b** *up*).

10 (**a** *flexion;* **b** *extension*) of the toes is a normal response to the plantar reflex.

11 To elicit a Babinski response, the examiner should stroke the (**a** *medial;* **b** *lateral*) aspect of the sole of the foot.

12 The scrotum should (**a** *elevate;* **b** *descend*) in a normal cremasteric response.

13 Resistance to neck (**a** *flexion;* **b** *extension*) may mean meningeal inflammation.

14 Pain upon straightening the knee with the hip and knee flexed is known as (**a** *Kernig's sign;* **b** *Chvostek's sign*).

Adult

15 Normal response to the jaw jerk in the adult is (**a** *no response;* **b** *quick closing of the jaw*).

16 The pouting reflex is (**a** *normal;* **b** *abnormal*) in the adult.

17 The grasp reflex is (**a** *normal;* **b** *abnormal*) in the adult.

Pediatric

18 Fanning of the toes is a/an (**a** *normal;* **b** *abnormal*) response to the Babinski reflex in the five-month infant.

19 The (**a** *Chaddock;* **b** *glabella*) reflex is evaluated in the same way as the Babinski.

Review Questions

True—False

Pediatric

____**20** The acoustic blink reflex should be routinely tested on all school age children.

____**21** A normal response to the tonic neck reflex at three months is the "fencer position."

____**22** The tonic neck reflex is normal in the eight-month-old infant.

____**23** Sustained ankle clonus is abnormal in an infant of any age.

____**24** Sucking facilitates the grasp reflex in the two-month-old infant.

____**25** The palmar grasp reflex should diminish after about three months.

____**26** The withdrawal reflex is elicited by pricking the soles of the feet of the infant.

____**27** The rooting reflex is an abnormal response in the neonate.

____**28** If the Moro reflex lasts more than four months, one should suspect a neurologic defect.

Matching
(Match the normal response with the appropriate reflex)

Part I

____29 Galant's reflex
____30 parachute reflex
____31 positive supporting reaction

a) when head is restrained, eyes turn in direction being turned
b) trunk turning to side of scratch
c) extension of legs with weight-bearing
d) extension of arms and legs when upper half of body is quickly lowered

Part II

____32 protective side-turning reflex
____33 Landau reflex

a) turning head to one side
b) flexion of hip, knee and ankle
c) lifting of head and extension of spine and legs

CRANIAL NERVE FUNCTION

Behavioral Objectives

The student will be able to:

1 answer in writing all *Review Questions*
2 state in writing the function of each of the 12 cranial nerves
3 state in writing the tests used in evaluating the function of each of the cranial nerves
4 assess the cranial nerve function of three adults and three children of varying ages and record the findings appropriately, according to the check list provided.

Learning Activities

Required

A *Read:*
   1 Alexander and Brown
   2 Bates
   3 *AJN* Programmed Instruction. "Patient Assessment—Neurological Examination, Part I"

B *View:* Blue Hill Series videotapes *Pediatric Examinations—The Neuromuscular System—School-Age Child* and *The Neuromuscular System—Infant;* and *Physical Assessment—Neurological*

C *Examine and record findings* related to assessment of the cranial nerve function of three adults and three children of varying ages.

CHECK LIST

Cranial Nerve Function

The following list should be filled in for each assessment of cranial nerve function required in the learning activities.

Sex______________
Age______________

Cranial Nerve Function	**Describe Response to Specific Tests**	**Evaluate Whether Response Is:**		
		Normal	**Abnormal**	**Questionable**
olfactory				
optic				
oculomotor				
trochlear				
trigeminal				
abducens				
facial				
acoustic				
glossopharyngeal				
vagus				
spinal accessory				
hypoglossal				

Review Questions

Matching

(Match the function of the cranial nerves with the letter of the appropriate cranial nerve)

_____1 hearing
_____2 tongue movement
_____3 sensation in pharynx

a) #8 acoustic
b) #2 optic
c) #12 hypoglossal
d) #10 vagus

_____4 vision
_____5 lateral deviation of the eye
_____6 jaw movement

a) #2 optic
b) #5 trigeminal
c) #6 abducens
d) #12 hypoglossal

_____7 sense of smell
_____8 inward movement of the eye
_____9 elevation of upper eyelid

a) #4 trochlear
b) #3 oculomotor
c) #2 optic
d) #1 olfactory

_____10 pupillary constriction
_____11 taste on anterior ⅔ of tongue
_____12 sensation in mandibular area

a) #7 facial
b) #3 oculomotor
c) #5 trigeminal
d) #4 trochlear

_____13 moving muscles of forehead
_____14 sensation in posterior tongue
_____15 movement of sternocleidomastoid

a) #9 glossopharyngeal
b) #7 facial
c) #11 spinal accessory
d) #3 oculomotor

True—False

_____16 The second cranial nerve may be tested by asking the patient to identify the smell of coffee.
_____17 If you ask the patient to clench his teeth, you are checking the trigeminal nerve.
_____18 Touching the side of the face with a fine wisp of cotton is a way of testing for facial nerve function.
_____19 If the patient is unable to hold his eyes tightly closed, you suspect a problem with the facial nerve.
_____20 Asking the patient to stick out his tongue is a way of evaluating the hypoglossal nerve function.
_____21 Hoarseness may indicate a problem related to the hypoglossal nerve.
_____22 Having the patient shrug his shoulders is a way of evaluating the eleventh cranial nerve.
_____23 Palate and uvula deviation could be due to a lesion of the vagus nerve.
_____24 If the patient is unable to show his teeth you may suspect paralysis of the facial nerve.
_____25 Testing the corneal reflex is part of the assessment of the trigeminal nerve.

____**26** Testing visual acuity is a way of testing the second cranial nerve.
____**27** If hearing loss is present, you might suspect a problem related to the eighth cranial nerve.
____**28** The visual field test should be done in all four quadrants.
____**29** Sustained nystagmus is normal in children under three months of age.
____**30** Vestibular function of the acoustic nerve should be part of every routine examination of children and adults.
____**31** The vibrating tuning fork should be heard longer via bone conduction than via air conduction.
____**32** In testing olfactory sense, it is important to test both nostrils at the same time.

SENSORY SYSTEM FUNCTION

Behavioral Objectives

The student will be able to:

1 answer in writing all *Review Questions*

2 state that evaluation of the sensory system is done by using the following stimuli:
- a) pain
- b) temperature
- c) light touch
- d) vibration
- e) position
- f) discrimination techniques

3 assess the sensory system function of three adults and three children of varying ages, and record the findings appropriately, according to the check list provided.

Learning Activities

Required

A *Read:*
- **1** Alexander and Brown
- **2** Bates
- **3** *AJN* Programmed Instruction. "Patient Assessment—Neurological Examination, Part II"

B *View:* Blue Hill Series videotapes *Pediatric Examinations—The Neuromuscular System—School-Age Child* and *The Neuromuscular System—Infant;* and *Physical Assessment—Neurological*

C *Examine and record findings* related to assessment of sensory system function of three adults and three children of varying ages.

CHECK LIST

Sensory System Function

The following list should be filled in for each assessment of sensory function required in the learning activities.

Sex______________
Age______________

Sensory System Function: Response to	Describe Response to Specific Tests	Evaluate Whether Response Is:		
		Normal	Abnormal	Questionable
pain				
temperature				
light touch				
vibration				
position				
discrimination techniques				

Review Questions

TRUE—FALSE

____1 In testing for primary sensation, it is essential that the face, trunk, arms, and legs be tested.

____2 The normal person can feel, but may not be able to localize the feeling response to superficial tactile sensations.

____3 It is most important to compare sensitivity side for side.

____4 Stereognostic sensation, graphesthesia, and texture discrimination are included in cortical and discriminating forms of sensation.

____5 Asking the patient to distinguish heads from tails on a coin by touch would be a way to test stereognosis.

____6 The stimuli used in testing the sensory system should be scattered to cover most of the dermatomes and major peripheral nerves.

____7 The test for extinction is done by simultaneously stimulating corresponding areas on both sides of the body and asking the patient where he feels the stimulation.

____8 The examiner should compare sensitivity in the proximal and distal portions of the extremities.

Pediatric

____9 The sensory system tests used on adults are reliable by the time the child reaches eight months of age.

ANSWER CHOICE

(Choose the correct answer in the parentheses)

10 Normal sensitivity to superficial tactile sensation is (**a** *the same;* **b** *not the same*) on all parts of the body.

11 The greatest sensitivity to vibration is found between (**a** *200–400 cycles/sec.;* **b** *50–100 cycles/sec.*).

12 Deep pressure pain is (**a** *routinely;* **b** *not routinely*) tested in all patients.

13 The average person can distinguish two separate stimuli on the two-point discrimination test on the fingertip when the stimuli are (**a** *one millimeter apart;* **b** *four to eight millimeters apart*).

14 Point localization requires that (**a** *only one point;* **b** *two points*) be used in the test.

Self-Evaluation Key

DEFINITIONS—CEREBRAL FUNCTION (p. 230)

1. D
2. G
3. A
4. J
5. L
6. I
7. E
8. B
9. M
10. O
11. N
12. K
13. H
14. F
15. C

REVIEW QUESTIONS—CEREBRAL FUNCTION (pp. 230–231)

1. T
2. T
3. F
4. T
5. T
6. F
7. F
8. F
9. T
10. F
11. F
12. T
13. T
14. F
15. T
16. T
17. T
18. T
19. T
20. T
21. T
22. T
23. F
24. T

REVIEW QUESTIONS—CEREBELLAR FUNCTION (p. 233)

1. T
2. T
3. T
4. T
5. T
6. T
7. T
8. T
9. F
10. T
11. F

DEFINITIONS—MOTOR SYSTEM FUNCTION (p. 235)

1. C
2. G
3. E
4. H
5. D
6. A
7. F
8. B

REVIEW QUESTIONS—MOTOR SYSTEM FUNCTION (p. 236)

1. T
2. F
3. T
4. F
5. T
6. T
7. T
8. T
9. F
10. T
11. T
12. T
13. T
14. T
15. a
16. a
17. b
18. a

REVIEW QUESTIONS—REFLEX ACTIONS (pp. 240–241)

1. a
2. a
3. b
4. b
5. a
6. a
7. a
8. a
9. b
10. a
11. b
12. a
13. a
14. a
15. b
16. b
17. b
18. a
19. a
20. F
21. T
22. F
23. T
24. T
25. T
26. T
27. F
28. T
29. b
30. d
31. c
32. a
33. c

REVIEW QUESTIONS—CRANIAL NERVE FUNCTION (pp. 243–244)

1. a
2. c
3. d
4. a
5. c
6. b
7. d
8. b
9. b
10. b
11. a
12. c
13. b
14. a
15. c
16. F
17. T
18. F
19. T
20. T
21. F
22. T
23. T
24. T
25. T
26. T
27. T
28. T
29. F
30. F
31. F
32. F

REVIEW QUESTIONS—SENSORY SYSTEM (p. 246)

1. T
2. T
3. T
4. T
5. T
6. T
7. T
8. T
9. F
10. b
11. a
12. b
13. b
14. a

additional references and materials

GENERAL BIBLIOGRAPHY

Adult

1 Prior, John, and Silberstein, Jack: *Physical Diagnosis.* 4th ed. St. Louis, C. V. Mosby Co., 1973.

2 Judge, Richard, and Zuidema, George: *Methods of Clinical Exam: A Physiologic Approach.* 3rd ed. Boston, Little, Brown and Co., 1974.

3 DeGowin, Elmer, and DeGowin, Richard: *Bedside Diagnostic Evaluation.* 3rd ed. New York, Macmillan Co., 1976.

4 Hudak, Carolyn M.; Lohr, Thelma; and Gallo, Barbara M.: *Critical Care Nursing.* 2nd ed. Philadelphia, J. B. Lippincott Co., 1977.

Pediatrics

1 Kempe, C. Henry; Silver, Henry K.; and O'Brien, Donough: *Current Pediatric Diagnosis and Treatment.* 3rd ed. Los Altos, Calif., Lange Medical Publications, 1974.

2 Barness, Lewis: *Manual of Pediatric Physical Diagnosis.* Chicago, Year Book Medical Publishers, Inc., 1972.

Obstetrics

1 Hellman, Louis, and Pritchard, Jack: *Williams Obstetrics.* 15th ed. New York, Appleton-Century-Crofts, 1976.

2 Romney, Seymour, et al.: *Gynecology and Obstetrics: The Health Care of Women.* New York, McGraw-Hill Book Co., 1975.

3 Taylor, E. S. (ed.): *Beck's Obstetrical Practice.* 9th ed. Baltimore, Williams and Wilkins, 1971.

SPECIFIC BIBLIOGRAPHY AND MATERIALS

Abdomen

G.I. Series: Physical Examination of the Abdomen
(Booklets, Parts I–V, Adult and Pediatric Series)
Richmond, A. H. Robins Co., 1972.

Breast

How to Examine Your Breast
16 mm film (6 minutes)
American Cancer Society, 219 East 42nd St., New York, N.Y. 10017, 1976.

Cardiovascular

1 Examination of the Heart (series of 5 pamphlets)
   I Data Collection: The Clinical History
   II Inspection and Palpation of Venous and Arterial Pulses
   III Inspection and Palpation of the Anterior Chest
   IV Auscultation
   V The Electrocardiogram
   American Heart Association, 44 East 23rd St., New York, N.Y. 10010, 1967.
2 Cardiac Auscultation, by Abe Ravin
   Audiotape cassettes (series of 6)
   Merck, Sharp and Dohme, Division of Merck and Co., Inc., West Point, Pa. 19486
3 Recommendations for Human Blood Pressure Determination by Sphygmomanometers (Booklet)
   American Heart Association, 44 East 23rd St., New York, N.Y. 10010, 1967.
4 Luisada, Aldo A., and Sainani, Gurmukh, S.: *A Primer of Cardiac Diagnosis.* St. Louis, Warren H. Green, Inc., 1968.
5 *Cardiac Auscultation*
   Videotape series
   Roche Laboratories, Division of Hoffman-LaRoche, Inc., Nutley, N.J. 07110.
6 Heart Sounds
   Audiotapes
   Roche Laboratories, Division of Hoffman-LaRoche, Inc., Nutley, N.J. 07110.
7 *Introduction to Arrhythmias*
   Slide series with tape
   Trainex Corp., P.O. Box 116, Garden Grove, Calif. 92641.

Chest and Lungs

The Chest: Its Signs and Sounds, by George Druger, M.D.
Text-tape packet
Humetrics Corp., 353 North Oak St., Inglewood, Calif. 90302.

Ear

1 Becker, Walter, et al.: *Atlas of Otorhinolaryngology and Bronchoesophagology.* Philadelphia, W. B. Saunders Co., 1969.
2 Anderson, B., M.D.; Buckingham, R. A., M.D.; Melloni, B. J.; and Holinger, P. H., M.D.: *Some Pathological Conditions of the Eye, Ear and Throat, An Atlas.* Chicago, Abbott Laboratories, 1977.

Eye

1 Butler, Patricia. "Physical Appraisal of the Eye and Vision." Pages 105–120 in *Physical Appraisal Methods in Nursing Practice.* Josephine Sana and Richard Judge (eds.) Boston, Little, Brown and Co., 1975.
2 Anderson, B., M.D.; Buckingham, R. A., M.D.; Melloni, B. J.; and Holinger, P. H., M.D.: *Some Pathological Conditions of the Eye, Ear and Throat, An Atlas.* Chicago, Abbott Laboratories, 1977.
3 Paton, David, M.D., and Hyman, Barry, M.D.: *Introduction to Ophthalmoscopy.* Kalamazoo, Mich., Upjohn Co., 1976.

Genitalia

1 *The Female Pelvic Examination*
Film
Indiana University Medical Center, Indianapolis, Ind. 46204.
2 Greenhill, J. P.: *Office Gynecology,* 9th ed. Year Book Medical Publishers, Inc., 1971.

Head, Face, and Neck

1 The Head (Number 2 of a series on variations and minor departures in newborn infants)
(Pamphlet)
Evansville, Ind., Mead Johnson Co., 1977.
2 *The Face* (I and II); *The Neck*
Films
CIBA Pharmaceutical Co., 556 Morris Ave., Summit, N.J. 07901.

Musculoskeletal (Spine and Extremities)

1 The Extremities, Parts I and II (Numbers 7 and 8 of a series on variations and minor departures in newborn infants)
(Pamphlets)
Evansville, Ind., Mead Johnson Co., 1976 (Part I), 1972 (Part II).
2 *Gait and Musculoskeletal Disorders*
Film
CIBA Pharmaceutical Co., 556 Morris Ave., Summit, N.J. 07901.
3 *Diagnosis of Congenital Dislocated Hip*
Film
CIBA Pharmaceutical Co., 556 Morris Ave., Summit, N.J. 07901.

Neurological

1 *Essentials of the Neurological Examination,* by Bernard J. Alpers and Elliott L. Mancall, 1971
Videotape
Smith, Kline and French Laboratories, 1500 Spring Garden St., P.O. Box 7929, Philadelphia, Pa. 19101.
2 Essentials of the Neurological Examination
(Booklet)
Philadelphia, Smith, Kline and French Laboratories, 1976.

Nose, Mouth, and Throat

1 Dental Symposium: *The Practitioner,* 214:337–356, March 1975.
2 The Mouth (Number 5 of a series on variations and minor departures in newborn infants)
(Pamphlet)
Evansville, Ind., Mead Johnson Co., 1969.
3 Anderson, B., M.D.; Buckingham, R. A., M.D.; Melloni, B. J.; and Holinger, P. H., M.D.: *Some Pathological Conditions of the Eye, Ear and Throat, An Atlas.* Chicago, Abbott Laboratories, 1977.
4 Smoking and Cancer
(Pamphlet)
Chicago, American Dental Association, 1972.
5 Seven Warning Signs of Gum Disease
(Pamphlet)
Chicago, American Dental Association, 1977.
6 Kerr, D. A.; Ash, M. M.; and Millard, H. D.: *Oral Diagnosis.* 4th ed. St. Louis, C. V. Mosby Co., 1974.
7 Scopp, Irwin: *Oral Medicine.* 2nd ed. St. Louis, C. V. Mosby Co., 1973.
8 Moss, Stephen J., (ed.): *Preventative Dentistry.* Cincinnati, Ohio, Proctor and Gamble, Crest Professional Services Div., 1972.
9 *Oral Lesions in Children and Adults*
Film (available on loan)
Wayne State University, 5980 Cass Ave., Detroit, Mich. 48202.
10 *Oral Cancer*
Film
American Cancer Society, 219 East 42nd St., New York, N.Y. 10017.

Skin and Lymphatic System

1 Skin Lesions Depicted and Defined: Part I—Primary Lesions; Part II—Secondary Lesions, by R. Caplan, M.D.; Alfred W. Kopf, M.D.; and Marion B. Sulzberger, M.D.
Slides with audiotapes (each 20 minutes)
Institute for Dermatologic Communication and Education, 2785 Jackson St., San Francisco, Calif. 94115, 1971.
2 *Common Skin Disorders in the First Year of Life,* by David L. Cramm, M.D.
Videotape (National Continuing Medical Education)
Roche Laboratories, Division of Hoffman-LaRoche, Inc., Nutley, N.J. 07110, 1975.
3 The Skin: Birthmarks (Numbers 1 and 4 of a series on variations and minor departures in normal infants)
(Pamphlets)
Evansville, Ind., Mead Johnson Co., 1976 (No. 1); 1972 (No. 4).